Researching User Perspectives on Community Health Care

Edited by

Bob Heyman

Reader in Health Sciences, Institute of Health Sciences,
University of Northumbria, UK

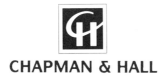

CHAPMAN & HALL

London · Glasgow · Weinheim · New York · Tokyo · Melbourne · Madras

Published by Chapman & Hall, 2–6 Boundary Row, London SE1 8HN, UK

Chapman & Hall, 2–6 Boundary Row, London SE1 8HN, UK

Blackie Academic & Professional, Wester Cleddens Road, Bishopbriggs, Glasgow G64 2NZ, UK

Chapman & Hall GmbH, Pappelallee 3, 69469 Weinheim, Germany

Chapman & Hall USA, One Penn Plaza, 41st Floor, New York NY 10119, USA

Chapman & Hall Japan, ITP-Japan, Kyowa Building, 3F, 2-2-1 Hirakawacho, Chiyoda-ku, Tokyo 102, Japan

Chapman & Hall Australia, Thomas Nelson Australia, 102 Dodds Street, South Melbourne, Victoria 3205, Australia

Chapman & Hall India, R. Seshadri, 32 Second Main Road, CIT East, Madras 600 035, India

Distributed in the USA and Canada by Singular Publishing Group Inc., 4284 41st Street, San Diego, California 92105

First edition 1995

© 1995 Chapman & Hall

Typeset in Palatino 10/12 by Saxon Graphics Ltd, Derby
Printed in Great Britain by St Edmundsbury Press, Bury St Edmunds, Suffolk

ISBN 0 412 49820 0   1 56593 300 1 (USA)

A catalogue record for this book is available from the British Library

Library of Congress Catalog Card Number: 94-68716

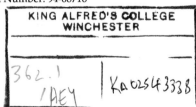
♾ Printed on permanent acid-free text paper, manufactured in accordance with ANSI/NISO Z39.48-1992 and ANSI/NISO Z39.48-1984 (Permanence of Paper).

To Ruth, Michael, Anna,
Daniel and Jess

Glendower: I can call spirits from the vasty deep.
Hotspur: Why, so can I, or so can any man; But will they come
when you do call for them?

Henry IV Part 1, Act III, Scene 1

Contents

Contributors

Joan E. Aarvold SRN, ONC, BSc, CertEd is a senior lecturer at the Institute of Health Sciences, University of Northumbria, specializing in health informatics and European health issues. She is a National Childbirth Trust antenatal tutor and has worked for 20 years in education and support for maternity service consumers. For the last seven years, she has been a lay representative on the Newcastle Health Authority Maternity Services Liaison Committee.

Geraldine S. Byrne RGN, BA, PhD worked for five years in medical/surgical nursing, and is now principal lecturer in nursing at the University of Hertfordshire. Her PhD, awarded by the University of Northumbria, focused on patient anxieties in accident and emergency departments.

Charlotte L. Clarke RGN, BA, MSc, PGCE worked as a nurse with the elderly for five years. She is now employed as a nurse teacher with Bede, Newcastle and Northumbria College of Health Studies. She is completing a PhD, based on her research into the needs of informal carers of elderly people suffering from dementia, at the University of Northumbria.

Jean Davies RGN, RM, MSc is a community midwife, working in Newcastle-upon-Tyne. She has been working with low-income women in an inner city area for over 10 years, has had wide experience teaching antenatal groups and has taught and written about matters relating to women and midwifery. She is currently working with the Northern Regional Maternity Survey Office on the 1993 Home Birth Study.

Nigel Davison RN, RMN, NDN, PgDip is a clinical specialist with responsibility for nursing development, particularly research into the organization and decision-making processes of community nurses.

Elizabeth Handyside BSc, MSc worked as a senior health promotion officer, with a special interest in HIV/AIDS, at York Health Authority and then as a researcher, evaluating HIV services in the area. She is about to begin another project, funded by the Northern Regional Health Authority and concerned with the sexual health of adults with learning difficulties, at the University of Northumbria.

Bob Heyman BA, PhD is a Reader at the Institute of Health Sciences, University of Northumbria and teaches social research methods and health psychology. He has researched social aspects of health for nearly 20 years and is a member of the Newcastle-upon-Tyne Local Medical Ethics Committee.

Sarah Huckle BA, MSc worked for three years on a research project involving the needs of adults with learning difficulties, at the Institute of Health Sciences, University of Northumbria, and is currently writing up her PhD. She is now working on a project which evaluates the impact of market forces on the provision of support services for children with special needs, at the University of Northumbria.

Mike Kingham BA, MSc, PGCE, NUJ Cert. is a Principal Lecturer, specializing in medical sociology, at the Institute of Health Sciences, University of Northumbria and is Programme Director for the Postgraduate Diploma/MSc Health Sciences. He has edited the British Sociological Association's Medical Sociology News, published research on the culture of drug use, and participated in the local and national AIDS initiatives. His current research interest is the historical representation of health and illness in cinema drama.

Tony Machin RMN, MSc, PGCE, RNT has a CPN background and has worked extensively with people with addiction problems. He is currently a nurse teacher with Bede, Newcastle and Northumbria College of Health Studies.

Susan J. Milner BA, PGD Health Education, RGN is Subject Leader in Health Promotion at the Institute of Health Sciences, University of Northumbria. During the last 17 years she has worked as a nurse and then as a health promotion specialist, finally as Regional Health Promotion Officer for the Northern Region.

Sarah Nettleton BA, MSc, PhD is a lecturer in social policy at the University of York. She has researched and published extensively in the area of sociology of health and illness.

Pauline Pearson RGN, RHV, BA, DipSocRes, PhD worked for many years as a health visitor and is currently Lecturer in Primary Care Nursing at the University of Newcastle. Her current research interests include teamwork in primary care and evaluation of service developments. Her PhD, on which her chapter is based, was undertaken at the Institute of Health Sciences, University of Northumbria.

Jan Reed RGN, BA, PhD is a lecturer in nursing at the Institute of Health Sciences, University of Northumbria. Her PhD looked at the assessment of older people in hospital wards. She is currently on secondment, funded by the Department of Health, and is working on a study which explores concepts of home and kinship in the care of older people.

Don Watson BA, MPhil, PhD is Professor and Head of the Institute of Health Sciences, University of Northumbria. He worked as a Psychologist in the health service before moving into higher education over 20 years ago. His research interests include individual differences, smoking behaviour and psychosocial aspects of community health care.

Acknowledgements

I would particularly like to thank Mike Kingham, from the University of Northumbria, for his advice and encouragement, Mick Carpenter, University of Warwick, for invaluable advice and suggestions, Joel Yoeli for considering the book from a professional perspective, Michelle Cowan for providing information about the French health system and Brian Bell for help with computer graphics. I would also like to thank all the health professional students who have taken the Postgraduate Diploma/MSc Health and Social Research and the MSc Health Sciences at the Institute of Health Sciences, University of Northumbria, over the last eight years, for sharing their ideas and experiences. Responsibility for views expressed rests entirely with the authors.

Introduction

Bob Heyman

RESEARCHING USER PERSPECTIVES ON COMMUNITY HEALTH CARE

> *The health service now has to learn to listen better to the public and be more guided by its wishes. It has to learn to trust them, to respect their opinions and respond to what they say. The people we serve should not be treated as mere passive recipients of care.*
> BRIAN MAWHINNEY (MINISTER OF HEALTH)
> ADDRESSING THE FEDERATION OF NHS TRUSTS,
> OCTOBER 1993

This book is about researching user perspectives on community health care. The problems of defining the slippery terms 'community', 'health', 'care', 'community health care' and 'perspectives', together with the rationale for researching user perspectives, will be discussed more fully in Chapters 1 and 2. The Introduction is intended only to highlight critical issues and to outline the scope, boundaries, limitations, origins and structure of the book.

User perspectives on health care are currently being given high political priority, at least rhetorically. Policy makers, purchasers and providers are turning to research as one way of finding out what the public want (NHSME, 1992). This double movement (prioritizing user perspectives and turning to research) promises boom times for social researchers in the health field. Instead of being condemned as 'unscientific' for not doing biomedical research, we are suddenly of interest to powerful figures in the medical and health service establishments and are finding research grants and consultancy easier to obtain.

The crest of a wave is a good position from which to ask awkward questions about what is going to happen next. Policy makers, purchasers and providers who have unrealistic expectations about the extent to which research can lead to more user-sensitive health care will become disillusioned if their expectations are not met. By providing a more critical analysis of the potential contribution of research, and its limitations, researchers may be able to minimize this disillusion, increasing the probability that research into user perspectives will continue to be supported.

A number of awkward questions about user perspectives and the role of research need to be asked. Why is there so much current concern with user perspectives? What does this concern tell us about the historical evolution of thinking about health services?

What are, and what should be, the relationships between lay and health professional perspectives, given that they mutually influence each other? For example, how should the health system respond to lay perspectives that are life-threatening (e.g. those of Dwight Harris, jailed in November 1993 for manslaughter after treating his diabetic daughter with complementary medicines)? How should the health system respond to the views of people such as child abusers, whose conduct is generally considered morally unacceptable? These examples, admittedly untypical, suggest that being 'guided' by user perspectives raises philosophical problems.

Why should research be chosen so frequently as the means to ensure that health care responds to user perspectives? Why, in Britain, are users of health services offered consultation but not participation or control?

Is social scientific research up to the job of accurately and sensitively articulating the varied perspectives of users? What are the power relationships between researchers, health professionals and users, and how do these relationships affect research outcomes? How far are researchers restrained by the need to retain health service customers? Conversely, to what extent do researchers exploit their evaluative power over health providers, for example looking for bad news because it makes good copy?

How far, and by what processes, can health care systems be influenced by research into user perspectives? Lynne Hunt, from Edith Cowan University, Western Australia, describes the 'pyjama game' that she plays with her young children. By involving them in a nightly choice about which pyjamas to wear, she avoids power struggles around the more important issue (to her) of what time they are to go to bed. Is user perspective research part of a national pyjama game?

This book will not attempt to answer such questions, but to illustrate the problems underlying them through discussions of recent research into user perspectives on health care.

Wicked problems

The idea of 'wicked problems' (Rittel and Weber, 1974; Kingsley and Douglas, 1991) is central to this book and to the rationale for taking user perspectives seriously. A 'wicked problem' is one which does not have an easy solution, because the advantages of all available approaches to the problem have to be balanced against inescapable disadvantages.

Dilemmas are thus central to the categorization of problems as wicked. However, the wickedness of a problem arises from the way it is perceived, rather than from the problem itself. A problem which one person finds easy may be 'wicked' to another. For example, Machin and Kingham, in Chapter 9, suggest that, for some health professionals, problem drinking is an easy problem solved by abstinence. For some drinkers, however, it is a wicked problem because they want to retain the benefits, to them, of heavy drinking, but do not want to suffer the adverse consequences.

The contributors to this volume agree with Kingsley and Douglas (1991) that the problems that community health care attempts to deal with are thoroughly wicked, particularly when long-term management is the best therapeutic response available. Some of the inescapable dilemmas faced by those with health needs, their carers and the wider society are outlined below.

What balance should be struck between minimizing risks for vulnerable people and maximizing their autonomy? This central dilemma surfaces in relation to home births (Chapter 5), residential care for the elderly (Chapter 7) and adults with learning difficulties (Chapter 10).

How should the moral obligation to help those in need be balanced against the requirement to avoid the creation of dependency? This problem is discussed in relation to sheltered accommodation for the elderly (Chapter 7).

How is responsibility for the support of people with disabilities to be apportioned between families, the local community and the wider society? For example, how can user choice be balanced against cost control? This question underlies all the chapters. It is one of the most important issues in current UK politics, as the New Right attempts to place as much responsibility as possible on families. How should the needs of those with health problems be balanced against those of their informal carers, an issue considered in relation to dementia (Chapter 8) and HIV (Chapter 12)?

How can the requirements of paid health work, e.g. division of labour, legalistic regulation and legitimate rights of health workers, be balanced against user need for choice, continuity, commitment and flexibility? For example, Chapter 12 describes the intense fear of an HIV patient that he could be let down if he became emotionally dependent on service providers who might become unavailable in the future when he most needed them.

How can the technical advantages of large specialist centres be weighed against the geographical and interpersonal advantages of smaller, more locally distributed health care institutions? This dilemma is discussed in Chapter 3 with respect to increased centralization of accident and emergency departments, in Chapter 5 in relation to home births and in Chapter 12 in connection with the advantages and disadvantages of specialist *versus* generic HIV services.

How can professional 'expert' status be reconciled with user-driven health care? This dilemma arises in all the chapters. For example, Chapter 6 discusses conflicts which occurred between health visitors and mothers as the mothers became more confident in the months following the birth of their first baby and began to feel that health visitors were not taking sufficient account of their views.

Such dilemmas, at the heart of community health care, cannot be 'solved' because they require that logically contradictory aims be achieved simultaneously. This is not an argument for fatalism. Appropriate and well resourced interventions can reduce the disadvantages arising from specific solutions to wicked problems. For example, if vulnerable people (e.g. the elderly, the mentally ill, those with learning difficulties) are encouraged to take risks in order to increase their autonomy, the risks can be reduced through training and provision of support. On the other hand, if people are institutionalized for their own safety, or to protect others, steps can be taken to maximize their autonomy within such settings. However, all available means of managing wicked problems will have costs as well as benefits and will produce varying outcomes which depend on circumstances in specific cases.

Because the dilemmas of community health care do not have correct solutions, they are bound to lead to differences of perspective between people with health problems, informal and formal carers, and within these groups. Decisions about the balance to be struck are inevitably affected by issues of power, interest and ideology (Saunders and Harris, 1990; Hugman, 1991). With wicked problems, better understanding of user perspectives can only be a first step towards making community health care more sensitive to their needs.

THE SCOPE OF THE BOOK

Origins

Since about 1980 the Institute of Health Sciences at the University of Northumbria has been increasingly involved in research into user perspectives on health care. This work has largely been initiated and carried out by health professionals, and seems to have been part of a wider wave of concern. User perspectives have been investigated at Northumbria in relation to discharge from hospital; accident and emergency departments; GP practices; health visiting; community midwifery, dentistry and physiotherapy; and community care for drug users, people with alcohol problems, the elderly, the mentally ill and adults with learning difficulties. Much of this work is represented in the book.

Although user perspectives have been a popular focus for this health professional research over the last decade, some changes of emphasis have occurred, perhaps reflecting historical shifts. Research concerned with medical treatment of specific conditions has gradually become less popular with our students (who are non-medical health professionals). Discharge planning first surfaced as a research topic in 1991, probably in response to the high profile recently given to community care. A new arrival in 1993, for better or worse, was research aimed at meeting the needs of purchasers and providers of health care. One project is attempting to classify physiotherapy problems, so that the provider can cost them. Another is trying to develop methods of assessing pressure sores that purchasers can use in evaluating care. A third project is attempting to develop information systems that can inform locality purchasing.

The heart of this book consists of chapters written by some of these researchers, reflecting on the methodological, professional and political implications of their work. Apart from the work on adults with learning difficulties (Chapter 10), the research was either service-commissioned (Chapters 4, 11 and 12), or initiated and carried out by health professionals themselves. The chapters selected are not intended to provide comprehensive cover of the field of community health care, but to give the reader an insight into some of the issues involved in researching user perspectives.

Boundaries

Current organizational issues in the health service are not a primary focus for the book, although they will be mentioned frequently. Indeed, one reviewer of the book proposal complained that it did not give enough prominence to 'sexy' issues such as purchaser/provider splits, fundholding and care plans. There are two reasons for this relative lack of emphasis on organizational issues. Firstly, most of the work on which the book is based was done in the 1980s and very early 1990s, predating many of the health service and community care reforms. The time-lags involved, although normal in academic research, illustrate one of the difficulties in generating research which can be used to guide the development of services. However, the chapters have all been written from the 'sharp end' of service delivery. The forms of health care considered are still intact, even if their organizational contexts have changed substantially, and the findings of the research are relevant to the future of community health care.

A second reason for not focusing on organizational issues is that users are primarily interested in the direct delivery of care. For example, most people don't even know if their GP practice is fundholding or not. It is not being argued that organizational matters are unimportant, only that user perspectives, like any other, give a limited 'picture' of health services, a picture which largely excludes organizational complexities. Greater awareness of user perspectives can, however, help health service purchasers and providers to focus on users' own priorities, on outcomes rather than delivery systems and outputs. Users can provide a valuable antidote to empty rhetoric, particularly that of policy makers and senior managers who are far removed from the actual provision of care.

This book will not provide a descriptive account of the health service and community care reforms. Nor will it help those looking for a text on how to research user perspectives. What the book does try to do is to give the reader an understanding, through examples, of the philosophical, theoretical, methodological, professional and political issues associated with research into user perspectives on community health care. The book is aimed at two main audiences: firstly, those working in the health field who have a practical interest in learning more about user perspectives; and secondly, the increasing number of students, mainly health professionals, undertaking research or higher education in community health care.

Inspection of the chapter headings will show a lack of respect for organizational boundaries that might be used to differentiate community health care from other forms of care. From a user perspective, distinctions between hospital and non-hospital care, primary and community care, health and social care are, at best, artificial. A chapter has been included on hospital care in accident and emergency departments (Chapter 3), on the grounds that both the causes and consequences of emergencies are often located in the community and require liaison with other agencies (e.g. to deal adequately with alcohol problems or family violence). Chapter 4 is concerned with primary care and its relationship to the local community.

The distinction between health and social care has also been ignored. There are cultural and ideological divides between health and social service workers (Dalley, 1993). But users do not split their needs up in order to match this division. A number of user groups, including the dementing elderly and their informal carers (Chapter 8), the mentally ill (Chapter 11) and HIV-positive people (Chapter 12), receive care from varying combinations of health, social and voluntary agencies.

Questions about defining community health care and differentiating it from 'non-community health care' will be considered in Chapter 1. For the purposes of this book, which is concerned with user perspectives, community health care will not be delineated organizationally, e.g. as non-hospital care, or geographically, e.g. as locally based care. Such distinctions reflect service, not user, priorities and reproduce divisions which users find irksome. Instead, health care will be considered to be 'community health care' if it is oriented to people with health problems **as members of communities**, and shows a concern for the human dimensions of health problems, for their economic, social, interpersonal, psychological and existential antecedents and consequences.

Common patterns

As editor, I have found it particularly interesting to discover commonalities running across the different health problems and care settings discussed in the book. These will be picked up later, and will merely be mentioned at this point.

Some of the main themes linking two or more chapters are:

- the gap between lay and professional perspectives on health and health care and the frequent failure of health professionals to recognize this gap;
- the sense which many people had of the local 'community' as hostile and dangerous;
- the importance to vulnerable users of long-term continuity of care;
- the ways in which users strategically manipulated the health system in order to increase their control over scarce caring resources, often at the price of increasing dependency;
- the tendency for projects to be suddenly killed off, or not get started, because they did not meet purchaser or provider priorities, despite research evidence that they were valued by users and were cost-effective.

Structure of the book

Chapters 1, 2 and 14 provide a general discussion of issues associated with researching user perspectives on community health care. Chapter 1 is devoted to definitional and conceptual problems. Chapter 2 debates the question 'Why study user perspectives on community health care?' and attempts to give both utilitarian and historical answers. Methodological issues are outlined in the last part of this chapter. Chapter 14 analyses current interest in user perspectives on community health care from a Foucauldian perspective, giving a more theoretical overview of the material which has been discussed in the book. Chapters 3–13 contain accounts of research into user perspectives in a variety of areas of community health care.

CHAPTER 1

Matters of definition

Bob Heyman

> *As is common with extended acquaintance with any task, topic or human being, Beatrice had an initial period of clear observation and detached personal judgment.... And then she became implicated.*
> BYATT, A.S. (1990) *POSSESSION: A ROMANCE*, P. 115

INTRODUCTION

It is hard to be against 'community', 'health' or 'care', but each term has a variety of meanings, leading to inevitable confusions which can sometimes be politically useful. The sections to follow discuss the concepts of 'community', 'health', 'care', 'community health care', 'users' and 'perspectives'. In preparation for these sections, the nature of definition itself will be briefly considered.

DEFINING DEFINITION

This section briefly introduces some concepts related to the process of definition itself, namely language games, the double hermeneutic and symbolic interaction. Definitional issues are particularly important with weasel words such as 'community', 'health' and 'care'.

Language games

Language games with 'community health care'

Wittgenstein's notion of language games has revolutionized our understanding of the process of definition. This revolution underpins social scientific approaches which focus on the interpretation of meaning, for example symbolic interactionism (Blumer, 1969).

When we attempt to define a term, it is natural to think that we are trying to find its essential meaning. However, language is a tool that we use in everyday life to achieve certain ends. To be useful, words need to have some flexibility. They come to have an evolving family of loosely connected meanings, associated through usage.

Kingsley and Douglas (1991, p. 22) discuss the difficulty in developing an 'unambiguous definition' of 'community'. The definitions which they cite include:

- communities of interest;
- geographical locations;
- a value system about care involving reduction of dependence on institutions and professionals, greater control of services by users and smaller localized care units;
- a mythical notion of self-sufficiency for all but acute and tertiary care.

The confusion which can arise from multiple meanings of the term 'community' has political advantages (Baldwin, 1993, p. 12). Governments concerned to limit public expenditure may wish the public to view community care in terms of a warm composite of the first three definitions while, in their expenditure decisions, operating on the basis of the fourth. Government and public can feel proud of their civilized policy of community care while passing the main care burden to unpaid family members (Dalley, 1988).

Language is a tool. The meanings of terms evolve because of their usefulness, not their definitional purity. There is a trade-off between precision and flexibility. Greater precision assists clarity of thought but narrows the range of contexts in which a term can be used. Broadening the meaning of a term increases its applicability but makes it more likely that language users will overlook important differences between entities with the same name and become confused.

The idea of language games, firstly, will be discussed in relation to the 'markets' in health and social care associated with the NHS and Community Care Act of 1990. It will be argued that the use of the term 'market' in these contexts stretches its meaning too far, creating confusion. Language games with the terms 'community', 'health' and 'care' will be discussed later in the chapter.

Language games with 'the market'

A striking example of a term whose meaning has been stretched so far that it is more confusing than useful is 'the market', a concept which is central to the philosophy of the New Right. Because the term is used in a variety of contexts, we should not expect to be able to discover a single essential meaning for 'the market'.

One central use of the term refers to a complex social arrangement which has six characteristics:

1. a tangible product (good or service) which can be clearly specified;
2. separation between providers and purchasers of that product;
3. large numbers of providers and purchasers operating independently;
4. maximized provider freedom concerning the means of production (e.g. deregulation);
5. consumers who are the ultimate purchasers and have to exchange their own scarce resources (usually money) for the product;
6. providers who compete to persuade individual consumers to purchase their product.

There is, currently, intense political debate about the advantages and disadvantages of pure markets in the above sense. Proponents argue that markets are the best way of giving consumers leverage, however indirect, over providers and so ensuring that it is in providers' interests to meet consumer needs as efficiently as possible.

Against this one (but very important) advantage, opponents of pure markets can cite numerous disadvantages. Pure markets are inherently unstable, going through cycles of boom (underproduction leading to higher prices) and bust (higher prices leading to overproduction, lower prices and reduced supply). They promote a culture of selfish individual-ism and short-termism. They encourage 'cherry-picking' from the most lucrative parts of a market. They erode the rights of workers who lack scarce skills, as labour costs are forced down through competition. They are 'blind' to the external effects of market activities, both good (e.g. the environmental benefits of public transport), and bad (e.g. the damaging effects on local communities of open-cast coal mining). The efficient oper-ation of markets requires that both providers and consumers should have similar access to information about products. However, in practice, providers are likely to have an informational advantage over consumers, particularly with complex 'products' such as health care.

During the 1980s the above debate has been uncritically transferred to social arrangements that are not pure markets. One muddle has been between privatizing a state industry and creating a market, even if the privatized firm has a near monopoly. Decisions of monopoly purchasers – for example, not to buy locally produced coal for electricity generation – have been given a misleading veneer of rationality because they appear to reflect impersonal 'market forces'. The converse of this muddle is the assumption that the state sector is necessarily less efficient because it is not a 'market'. For example, local authorities have been compelled to spend most of the money provided for community care in the private and voluntary sectors, on the dubious grounds that the latter are inherently better at delivering efficient, high quality services.

The NHS and Community Care Act (1990) set up a 'managed' rather than a 'free' market. The system contains strong central control, as seen, for example, in the planned replacement of regional health authorities by offshoots of the NHS Management Executive (NHSME) in 1996. Commercial rhetoric, associated with the original planning of the reforms during the 1980s, has been softened in the changed political climate of the early 1990s. For example, 'buyers' have become 'purchasers' and then, sometimes, 'commissioners' (Butler, 1994, p. 22). Nevertheless, the idea that competition will improve the efficiency and quality of health services is central to the reforms. The most recent 'business plan' for the NHS (NHSME, 1993a) requires a shift in emphasis from maintaining a 'steady state' towards purchasing and the internal market (Appleby *et al.*, 1994, p. 46–47).

Use of the term 'market' to describe the present structure of health care requires the term to be stretched in two ways. Firstly, 'consumers' of health care are also its 'producers' (Stacey, 1976), unless, fatally, we confound health with health care and so 'commodify' health (Carpenter, 1994). Secondly, users have no purchasing power over the provision of state health services in the internal market. Power is exercised on their behalf by fundholding GPs, district health authorities and local authorities, themselves subject to centrally imposed financial constraints (Ranade, 1994, p. 71).

Even Le Grand and Bartlett (1993), who wish to defend the idea of quasi-markets for health and social care, concede this point. They note that 'ironically' one major change associated with the NHS and Community Care Act, the elimination of the residential care allowance in social security payments, has removed one of the few areas of direct choice available to consumers, as these payments are now under the control of care managers (p. 5). However, lack of consumer choice is fundamental to cash-limited services funded by the state (Mullen, 1991). For example, the new system of formal assessment of elderly people, required before they can receive places in care homes, is giving those who are turned down less choice than they had before 1993 (Counsel and Care, 1994).

Since purchasers buy care on behalf of users, they are not themselves subject to competition. The tag 'internal market' may prevent people from asking questions about purchaser motivation and capability. Le Grand and Bartlett (1993) assert: 'However, it might be thought that a lack of competition among **purchasers** would present fewer problems for quasi-markets, at least from a user perspective' (p. 20).

But they give no analysis of why this should be the case. Split-off purchasers may have less vested interests in the provision of particular forms of care and, therefore, more freedom to take account of user perspectives, a significant potential advantage.

On the other hand, purchaser/provider splits enlarge the distance between purchasers and users, increasing the danger of purchaser ignorance. And they create the potential for intergroup conflicts between purchasers and providers. Sociologists and social psychologists emphasize, to a greater extent than economists, the power of group identification (Tajfel, 1982) and organizational culture. Communication breakdowns and disputes occur frequently when different cultures interact. Early work on the impact of the 1990 NHS and community care reforms suggests that purchaser/provider tensions may be developing, since purchasers appear happier than providers with the contracting process (Appleby *et al.*, 1994, p. 39).

Purchaser/provider splits create knotty and expensive contracting problems (Bartlett and Harrison, 1993, p. 71). Precise contracts tend to be too rigid, while vaguer ones allow providers ample scope to interpret their terms in ways that suit their own interests. Purchasers have found the monitoring of contracts problematic because providers, on whom they depend for such information, have tended to supply late, poor quality data (Appleby *et al.*, 1994, p. 42).

Even if good quality outcome data can be obtained, the relationship between this 'evidence' and purchasing policy will be unavoidably problematic, political and dependent on value judgements (McKeown *et al.*, 1994, p. 19). For example, QALYS (quality adjusted life years) have been criticized (Carr-Hill, 1989) for providing spurious numerical objectivity. QALYS contain concealed value judgements about the relative 'costs' of morbidity and mortality, and about risk tolerance and time trajectories (e.g. the subjective 'cost' to an individual of an increased risk of morbidity or mortality in the distant future).

In so far as purchasers ignore provider interests, and attempt to maximize competition, they may generate health systems which are fragmented and unstable, with plummeting morale among health service workers. Such systems are unlikely to be sensitive to user perspectives. To avoid creating such systems, purchasers need to develop symbiotic, long-term relationships with providers, in 'relational markets' (Ranade, 1994, p. 73), compromising the split from providers.

Purchaser/provider splits are exacerbated by purchaser/purchaser splits, since 'health' care is purchased by district health authorities and GP fundholders, while 'social' care is purchased by local authorities. However, the split between health and social care is entirely organizational. It is not based on the experiences or needs of 'consumers', i.e. people with health problems and their informal carers (Hunter, 1994, p. 17).

The indivisibility of 'health' and 'social' problems, from users' perspectives, stands out as a theme in the research chapters in this book. Patients in accident and emergency departments are as much concerned with the social consequences of the accident or emergency as with the medical problem itself (Chapter 3). Poor people see their health problems as caused by social deprivation and in need of socioeconomic and environmental solutions (Chapter 4). Midwifery services are over-medicalized and the wider needs of mothers-to-be and their families have been neglected (Chapter 5). Alcohol problems are as much social and interpersonal as psychological and medical (Chapter 9). It appears to be almost random whether the lead carer for dementia sufferers (Chapter 8) or people with mental health problems (Chapter 11) comes from health or social agencies. People with mental health problems account for their problems using a mixture of psychological and social explanations, the latter becoming more important as their mental health improves (Chapter 11). HIV-positive people can experience problems when they try to be referred from health to social agencies (Chapter 12).

Coordination problems, boundary disputes and conflicts between health and local authority purchasers are a danger within this purchaser/purchaser split system. Moreover, the ground rules in the two subsystems differ significantly (Carpenter, 1994, ch. 5). Local authority 'social' care is means-tested, severely cash-limited (because it has a lower profile with voters) and heavily biased towards private sector and voluntary provision. 'Health' care is only means-tested at the margins, e.g. for prescriptions, has not suffered the kinds of cuts in financial support which have been imposed on local authorities and is largely provided by state sector organizations such as health trusts. Local and district health authority boundaries often do not match. Organizational differences are emerging, as DHAs aggregate purchasing while social service department budgets are devolved to smaller units (Wistow, 1994, p. 32).

Disputes over whether a particular form of care is 'health' or 'social', a false, organizationally driven distinction, are already emerging. For example, the NHS is opting out of long-term geriatric care, despite evidence of the efficiency and quality of NHS nursing homes, leaving people to rely on largely private, means-tested provision (Henwood, 1992). Early discharge from hospital, a financial priority for purchasers and providers of acute health services, is not necessarily important to social service departments, who purchase community services on which early discharge often depends (Wistow, 1994, p. 30). Attempts to provide long-term housing for the seriously mentally ill have been frustrated because of coordination problems between the Department of Health and other agencies (House of Commons Health Committee, 1994). In this book, Milner and Watson (Chapter 13) report that a new district health authority purchaser stopped funding a support scheme for self-help groups because they classified it as a social services responsibility and not one of their priorities.

The divide between health and social care predates the NHS and Community Care Act of 1990. However, the withdrawal of the NHS from social care, as seen for example in earlier discharge from hospital and the closure of long-term geriatric facilities, has made lack of coordination between health and social services potentially more damaging than it might have been in the past. Boundary issues can be expected to cause continuing problems as the new 'market-driven' NHS continues to divest itself of 'social' care. And initiatives that attempt to integrate health and social care, such as joint health/local authority planning, will have to attempt to bridge the organizational and cultural divide (Dalley, 1993) which separates these two types of purchaser. It is easy to underestimate the difficulty of this task.

There are excellent purchasers, attempting to maximize service quality and cooperating as well as they can with other agencies. But, in the absence of democratic or user participation or control and of agencies which can take a strategic overview of the health, social, environmental and economic needs of localities, quality depends on the personal qualities and public service idealism of individuals, not on market forces. Purchasing that is sensitive to the needs of the users discussed in this book requires well paid, middle class managers, often entrenched in service bureaucracies, cultures and career structures, to be long-term 'champions' (DOH, 1990, p. 17) of people who may be poor, stigmatized, chronically ill, inarticulate and unskilled in manipulating the welfare state. Examples of the inevitable problems which arise when health professionals make decisions 'on behalf of' users, without any checks or balances, are given below.

In the development of alternatives to residential care for adults with learning difficulties, district health authority purchasers have frequently favoured NHS trusts (in many cases, the old mental handicap hospitals) over social services, regardless of their suitability, because of professional rivalries (Collins, 1993). Provider trusts, according to Collins, have often had monopoly power and have pursued 'commercial' interests at the expense of users. Some purchasers have had no experience in the field of learning difficulties. Some have sought the cheapest solutions, regardless of quality, perhaps to enhance performance-related pay. They have frequently imposed detailed contracts that inhibit flexibility and user choice.

Problems have arisen with purchasing decisions which care managers make 'on behalf of' clients. A speaker at the 1993 Social Services conference stated that social workers' prejudices against clients whom they perceived as difficult were 'camouflaged in the language of assessment' (*Guardian*, 29/10/93).

The assumption that GPs will necessarily act in the interests of patients can also be questioned. For example, fundholding GPs kept back about £50 000 per practice in their first year (*Guardian*, 28/2/94), with the biggest savings sometimes occurring in regions with the worst waiting lists, e.g. NE Thames. Although doctors will not profit personally, they may spend this money to meet their own priorities rather than those of patients. Doctors have also been criticized for overprescribing as a substitute for spending more time talking to patients, although there are many examples of good practice (HMSO, 1994).

Burgess (1993), in a small qualitative study of patients waiting for hip replacements, found that some criticized their doctors for slowness in referring them and for failing to act as advocates when they were faced with long delays. As one patient said of her GP: 'He's opted out. He won't have anything to do with hospital waiting lists.' Other doctors were seen as effectively lobbying for their patients. The essential point for the present discussion is that, in the current 'internal market', patients have to rely on GPs and have no purchasing power of their own.

Three chapters in this book discuss projects that came to an abrupt halt, or didn't get started, through lack of support by those in authority, even though research had shown that they met user needs. The community midwifery project described in Chapter 5 was discontinued (admittedly before the implementation of purchaser/provider splits), despite evidence of clinical as well as user satisfaction benefits. The self-help support project considered in Chapter 13 was killed off by the newly established purchaser because it was not one of their priorities, although research evidence showed that it met user needs and was cost-effective. Chapter 4 discusses the rejection by an FHSA of proposals made by residents of a deprived estate to establish a combined community, health, leisure and welfare centre which they would 'own'.

These projects had two characteristics that may explain their failure. They were directed at the needs of socially disadvantaged groups and they required considerable power-sharing by health professionals.

The Minister of Health's rather desperate moral appeal to health service trusts to take more account of public views, quoted at the beginning of the Introduction, illustrates the shortcomings of describing the reformed NHS as a market. The whole point of a market is that providers **have** to take account of user views if they are to stay in business.

The argument is not that purchasers should not be split from providers, only that calling the reformed system a 'market' stretches the meaning of the term too far. As a result, careful analysis of the roles, interests and power relationships of purchasers, providers and users is avoided. The 1990 NHS and community care reforms, in so far as they do generate markets, create competition to please health service purchasers, not competition to meet the needs of 'consumers'.

Meanwhile, the public service ethos is being eroded as the trappings of market culture, including large pay increases for senior managers, competitiveness, secrecy and, occasionally, quasi-corruption are being enthusiastically adopted by some. The problem for the present Conservative government is that it cannot curtail the huge expansion in trusts' management costs, including self-awarded pay increases, without compromising its 'free market' rationale.

The role of user perspectives in developing community health care needs to be considered in the context of an 'internal market' which has ceded users little leverage over the care purchased on their behalf. Purchasers are not accountable to users, either directly or through democratic processes. The present system ultimately relies, ironically, on purchasers' public service idealism.

Symbolic interaction

The use of language is more than a game. Language reflects and shapes our choices about how to approach situations (e.g. choosing to view the health service as a market). Since social situations are symbolically constructed (Blumer, 1969), there will always be the potential for participants to generate conflicting role definitions. Such conflicts are inevitable in rapidly changing, pluralistic societies. It will be argued below that they are particularly endemic in relationships between purchasers, providers and users of community health care.

Where participants do not agree about the definition of the situation, four kinds of outcome are possible. Firstly, the participants may not realize that their definitions are contradictory. For example, Heyman and Huckle (1993a) found that some adults with learning difficulties would have liked to visit friends but were afraid to ask their parents. Their parents believed that they did not want to visit because they never asked. By not recognizing the person's need, informal carers, mostly women with heavy family commitments, were able to avoid taking up yet another responsibility.

Secondly, differences in symbolic definition of the situation may be recognized but glossed over. The flexibility of language permits the same terms to be used with different meanings, sidestepping conflict. This 'diplomatic' function of language will be discussed below in relation to analysis of the term 'community' (Cohen, 1985).

Thirdly, participants may try to negotiate, implicitly or explicitly, in order to make their definitions of the situation more compatible. Negotiation is not necessarily a mutual process of give and take and is affected by differences in material and definitional power. For example, Byrne, in Chapter 3, discusses the way in which nurses in accident and emergency departments used induction rituals to define entrants as 'patients' and ensure compliance. One of the most effective ways for health professionals to maintain their own power is to persuade the public to adopt their perspectives (Hugman, 1992).

Fourthly, there may be more or less open conflict in which the participants recognize incompatibility in their definitions of the situation, although not necessarily in direct communication. For example, Handyside (Chapter 12) found that some HIV-positives rejected local HIV services and were prepared to travel considerable distances to obtain support which they felt better met their needs.

Through research, it is possible to explore relationships between the perspectives of users, formal and informal carers. Chapters 3, 6, 7, 8, 10 and 12 explore aspects of these relationships.

The double hermeneutic

Hermeneutics is the study of meaning. The concept of the **double hermeneutic** (Habermas, 1984) reminds us that social scientists concerned with meaning have a double difficulty. The meanings which they study will themselves be shifting, variable and context-specific. But, to understand these meanings, the social scientist has to develop a technical vocabulary that allows them to be classified. This technical language is subject to the same vagaries as that of the people being studied. Different social scientists use terms such as community health care in various ways. The terms come to have a family of meanings, and usage depends on context.

Our everyday use of language is geared towards action, and so combines value orientation with description. The technical language employed must allow the social scientist to describe differences in orientation to the same phenomenon clearly. This will normally require the invention of neutral terms, which themselves are bound to become problematic as they acquire a variety of connotations. For example, in this book, the term 'user' has been given neutral status. A user can be a 'patient', 'client', 'consumer' or 'citizen', each term implying a different orientation to the relationship between users and health systems.

Such terms inevitably have their own hermeneutic problems. The term 'user', for example, implies a split between users and providers of health care, a split that arises out of the way in which, in western cultures, we tend to think about health 'services'. But, as already pointed out, users of health services can be seen as the primary producers of their own health (Stacey, 1976).

Social scientists have used 'locality' (Day and Murdoch, 1993) as a neutral term which avoids the assumption, implicit in the terms 'neighbourhood' and 'community', that the locality is a familiar, friendly place. This assumption may be particularly misleading for people with disabilities. Some elderly people living alone (Chapter 7) and adults with learning difficulties (Chapter 10) view the locality as a hostile, dangerous place.

Heyman and Huckle (Chapter 10) gave the term 'hazard' moral neutrality. The same hazard could be seen by adults with learning difficulties and their carers as a risk to be calculated (morally positive), or a danger to be avoided (morally negative). People managing practical problems associated with learning difficulty did not themselves think neutrally. For them, hazards were always risks or dangers.

Researchers have to take great care to unravel variations in actors' meanings, and to avoid assimilating them to their own perspectives. This will usually require qualitative methods, at least in the preliminary phase of the research.

PATIENTS, CLIENTS, CONSUMERS, CITIZENS AND USERS

Users and potential users of community health care may be viewed as 'patients', 'clients', 'consumers' or 'citizens'. These four terms can be located on a continuum in terms of an implicit balance of power between providers and users of services. Patients passively surrender control over both means and ends. Clients control ends, but are expected to defer to providers' greater expertise with respect to means. Consumers decide about both ends and means, influencing provision indirectly through their purchasing power. Citizens are the primary producers of their own health and have direct power over service provision, e.g. through self-help groups, democratic control or representation on the bodies that manage formal care.

The term 'user' will be employed to imply neutrality about power relationships. Users may be both people with health problems and their informal carers, but health professionals often have to deal with conflicts between the wishes and needs of these two parties (see Chapters 8, 10 and 12). The meaning of 'user' must also be stretched to include potential users who would use services if the need arose and disaffected non-users who would use services if they were different.

The concepts of 'patient', 'client' and 'consumer' are familiar in our culture and need little further discussion. Each locks into a wider system of belief. Patients are part of the medical model and are expected to obey doctors' instructions.

The term client has connotations of a legal adviser and is used in a wide range of caring contexts, e.g. client-centred psychotherapy (Rogers, 1951) and social work. A client has more legitimate 'say' over what he or she should do. In a legal context, a client may hire and fire a legal adviser, specify objectives and reject advice, but should do so with caution, given the lawyer's expertise.

In the public sector, UK users have very limited choice, if any, about the kinds of formal care that they may receive. Nevertheless, the concept of 'client' does convey the greater degree of active participation normally found in community health care compared with acute medicine. People with health problems and their informal carers provide so much of the input into community health care that they come to see themselves as being in control, even if health professionals do not agree.

The concept of 'consumer' locks into the ideology of the free market, through the idea that recipients of health care can be empowered by giving them choice about which services to purchase. The 'fittest' services which best meet a 'market need' should survive. The problems with applying the metaphor of the market to health care have already been analysed in the discussion of language games, and will be picked up in Chapter 2, when 'consumerism' will be considered.

Citizens, in contrast to consumers, have both rights and obligations (Turner, 1993, p. 3) to participate in the collective provision of services. This concept has no similarity to the 'citizen's charters', promoted at one time as the central tenet of 'Majorism'. Citizen's charters, including the Patient's Charter of 1991, simply stress consumer rights, e.g. redress for complaints, but do not give citizens any voice in the provision of services (Plamping and Delamothe, 1991). The charters appear to be popular with the public and, if effective, will provide useful regulatory consumer protection. But they do not give users any control over the system, either indirectly through consumer purchasing power or directly through citizenship and community participation.

Citizenship implies involvement by users of the health system in decisions about the provision of services, and thus contrasts with consumerism (Potter, 1988). During the period of Conservative government that began in 1979, community participation in public services has been significantly weakened in Britain, as services have been increasingly managed by quangos, e.g. health trusts, appointed politically by central government. The recent replacement of regional health authorities by outposts of the NHSME will increase central control, encourage secrecy and silence local voices yet further.

Genuine power sharing is one way out of the impasse of an internal market which gives users no systematic 'voice'. It will be discussed in the context of 'empowerment' in Chapter 2.

WHAT IS A COMMUNITY?

'Community' in modern societies

The term 'community' has multiple shades of meaning. Baldwin (1993, p. 31) claimed that the number of definitions had increased to over 200 by the 1980s!

Cohen (1985) argues that, in the modern world, structural communities marked by clear physical boundaries, e.g. villages, have been replaced by symbolic communities. These are defined by perceived similarities, which give members a sense of having something in common and of being differentiated from the rest of society. But such communities do not have physical boundaries. In modern usage, we talk about the 'gay community', the 'Jewish community' or the 'scientific community'. This usage is a good example of a language game because it bears only a family resemblance to its meaning in relation to structural communities.

In this modern usage, 'community' can be distinguished from 'locality' (Day and Murdoch, 1993). For many people, their locality is merely the area in which they live and is not a symbolic community. 'Locality care' would attract less public support than 'community care', but is, perhaps, a more realistic title.

Cohen makes two important points about symbolic communities. Firstly, the symbols which unite communities have a diplomatic vagueness that allows differences to be managed without conflict. For example, active members of a Jewish community might define 'Jewishness' in terms of religion, Zionism, a common history of persecution or the secular tradition. The same symbol can have different meanings with only a family resemblance, but can still unite members of the community.

Cohen's second point is that communities develop ways of maintaining differentiation from the outside world. This may be done through overt resistance or, with more subtlety, through syncretism, incorporating alien influences and transforming them to fit in with the values of the community.

An illustration of the modern sense of community, and its fragility, is given below in relation to a 'community' response to a toxic waste dump in a residential area. 'This [a blockade of the side gates] was the foundation for a real community ... if you didn't have anything else to talk about, there was always the site.... In a sense we're victims of our own success.... To be frank, things are a lot quieter now' (*Guardian*, 6/11/92).

'Community' in community health care

In community health care, the 'community' seems often to stand simply for the world outside institutions, for example when it is said that long-stay patients are being returned 'into' the community. However, it is instructive, applying Cohen's ideas, to reverse this perspective and consider health professionals as a community (or a number of communities). This does not imply that they hold identical views, only that they share a family of common experience and symbols, for example associated with belonging to the NHS.

Strauss and Corbin (1988) argue that several factors, including professional training, membership of formal health care organizations and repeated work-related contact with ill people, lead health professionals to intellectualize illness. Lay people are more concerned with the meaning of illness in their own daily lives. 'Their worlds are not the professional's world and *vice versa*' (Strauss and Corbin, 1988, p. 42).

Mutual misunderstanding is the likely result, often magnified by cultural differences associated with gender, ethnicity, social class and age in rapidly changing, pluralistic societies. Such misunderstandings were found in all the research discussed in this book, and are summarized in Chapter 2.

Communities, as Cohen emphasizes, define their symbolic essence *vis à vis* non-members. The term which health professionals seem to use for the out-group is 'the community'. It is easy to assume that non-health professionals have characteristics associated, however mythically, with traditional village communities, for example, psychological identification with the locality, solidarity with its residents.

Health professional usage of the term 'the community' to refer to the rest of society can be compared with that of the police. As we were counselled by the police in *The Real Inspector Hound* (Stoppard, 1970): 'The public is advised to stick together and make sure none of their number is missing' (p. 29).

Nettleton, in Chapter 14, makes a similar point, from a Foucauldian perspective, when she argues that communities are 'constructed', i.e. defined as conceptual entities, by forms of health care and social management.

Defining 'the community' as a place which institutionalized people can be moved to has the odd implication that health institutions are not part of 'the community' and thus reinforces the sense that health professionals are a community *vis à vis* the rest of the population. Research into user perspectives can be seen, in part, as an attempt by health professionals to break down the barriers of their own community, in order to understand the strange world outside.

WHAT IS HEALTH?

In relation to community health care, a broad definition of health is required, encompassing not just the absence of disease but also positive concepts of health and ways of coping with ill health. Broad definitions, inescapably, involve implicit or explicit value judgements. For example, one of the main attempts to define and classify the wider implications of health problems objectively has been the International Classification of Impairments, Disabilities and Handicaps (WHO, 1980).

Impairment is defined (my emphasis) as: 'any loss or **abnormality** of psychological, physiological or anatomical structure or function' (p. 47). Disability is defined as: 'any restriction or lack (resulting from impairment) of ability to perform an activity in the manner or range **considered normal** for a human being' (p. 143). Handicap is defined as: 'a disadvantage for a given individual, resulting from an impairment or a disability, that limits or prevents the fulfilment of a **role that is normal** (depending on age, sex, and social and cultural factors) for that individual' (p. 183).

The conservative assumption implicit in the WHO system, that what is normal in a society is also desirable, is arbitrary and dubious. There are problems in even deciding what is normal in concrete cases (Cicourel, 1973), especially in the socially esoteric situations encountered by people with disabilities and their informal carers. For example, is it normal for informal carers to devote their lives to caring for dependent relatives or to pass responsibility to the state? Is it normal for vulnerable people to face hazards in order to become more integrated into the community?

Szasz (1970) argues that definitions of health implicitly or explicitly involve some notion of the good life. No universal blueprint is possible because balances must be struck between irreconcilable alternatives, between individual freedom and equality, change and continuity, controlling nature and living in harmony with the natural world. Some of these choices can be made by individuals – e.g. not to smoke – but some can only be made collectively – e.g. to cut traffic pollution.

Professionals cannot claim exclusive expertise in defining health. Because users of community health services define health and health needs in their own ways and arrive at their own compromises, it is essential that they are given some control over the specification of the objectives of care.

WHAT IS CARE?

As with 'community' and 'health', there are a family of meanings associated with the term 'care', and it is important to consider the diplomatic function of shifts and ambiguities in meaning. Thomas (1993) discusses the extensive, mostly feminist, sociological literature and analyses care in terms of variations on seven dimensions:

- the social identity of the carer (e.g. wives, nurses);
- the social identity of the care recipient (e.g. children, people with disabilities);
- the interpersonal relationship between giver and receiver of care (e.g. familial, paid professional);
- the nature of care (e.g. emotional, practical);
- the social domain in which care is located (e.g. public, domestic);
- the economic character of the care relationship;
- the institutional setting in which care is delivered (e.g. home, hospital).

Two distinctions will be briefly discussed below, between 'caring for' and 'caring about' and between formal and informal care. Greater awareness of user perspectives may help health providers and purchasers to remember that 'care' can have many different meanings, since users will be sensitive to the reality of care rather than its labelling.

Caring for and caring about

Dalley (1988) analyses the minefield of confusion surrounding use of the term 'care', particularly the distinction, also made by other writers, between 'caring for' and 'caring about'.

Caring for involves looking after another person. Caring about is concerned with feelings for another person. In our society, Dalley argues, the two are conflated and are assumed to be 'natural' to women through the role of mother and its extension, e.g. the care of elderly relatives. Women who are reluctant to care for a relative may be stigmatized as not caring about that person, resulting in 'compulsory altruism'. This view is consistent with a New Right political position that seeks to minimize the responsibility of the state for providing for the needs of individuals. Conversely, lack of a distinction between caring for and caring about can lead to the assumption that those who care for a person (e.g. health workers) must care about that person.

Formal and informal care

James (1992) defines care as involving the combination of organization and physical and emotional labour. She argues that the notion of care as employed by health professionals is derived from its usage in family care, e.g. parents caring for children. But aspects of family care such as flexibility, provision of a wide range of care by a small number of carers and long-term personal commitment cannot readily be reproduced in formal care settings, even hospices.

A major difference arises from the complex division of labour in health care. Health professionals in a variety of settings, including the hospice studied by James, are now trying to develop an interdisciplinary 'team' approach to improve coordination, flexibility and involvement with individual patients. James felt that the team approach, although central to the treatment philosophy of the hospice movement, did not really improve emotional care.

However, it should not be assumed that paid care is necessarily inferior to unpaid care (Ungerson, 1990; Walmsley, 1993). The emotional quality of informal care is inevitably variable, and often fragile. Some elderly people may not wish to become dependent on their offspring. For younger disabled people, residential care may offer their only opportunity to leave home, given parental anxiety about independent living (see Chapter 10). A choice of options, including different combinations of paid and unpaid care, is needed.

WHAT IS COMMUNITY HEALTH CARE?

Defining community health care

Since this book is about user perspectives, an organizationally driven definition of community health care is inappropriate, as argued in the Introduction. Users experience health problems holistically. The health issues considered in the research chapters have inter-related medical, psychological, interpersonal, social and economic components.

Defining community health care organizationally, e.g. as care taking place outside large institutions, reproduces splits which users find irksome. It reinforces the notion that institutions such as hospitals are, somehow, not 'in' the community and entails the prejudgement that institutional care is necessarily bad. Similarly, as argued above in relation to purchasing, the split between health and social care creates arbitrary, organizationally driven fissures.

Community health care, from a user perspective, will be defined as care in any organizational or geographical context that treats people as members of communities and so is oriented to the human aspects of health problems. For example, hospital-based accident and emergency services that take account of patients' anxieties and wider social concerns should be considered as community health care, while the narrowly medical approach described in Chapter 3 should not.

The distinction between community and 'non-community' health care cannot be drawn precisely, only in terms of a 'family' of related characteristics, outlined below, some or all of which will be found in any particular example. Community health care:

- is oriented towards promotion of health, prevention of long-term health problems and amelioration of the human consequences of such problems, rather than towards cure;
- is associated with a critical attitude towards institutional, bureaucratic delivery of care;
- attempts to utilize and work with community resources, principally the family.

The first characteristic of community health care is that it is orientated towards the behavioural, psychological, social, lifestyle and economic antecedents and consequences of health problems, rather than just towards cure. Its main foci are health promotion and the prevention and management of chronic illness, which has a greater impact than acute illness on the lives of sufferers and their families (Strauss and Corbin, 1988). Such care requires community health professionals to confront the issue of defining normality and the value judgements that this entails.

A second characteristic of community health care is that it is associated with a reaction against the institutionalization of care, which is seen to disempower users. For example, Kirkham (1989) found that the power of mothers to influence the birth process increased successively between hospitals, GP units and their own homes. Women giving birth at home took more clinical decisions (e.g. when to have membranes ruptured) than midwives did in most consultant unit labours.

The advantage of decentralized community services, in terms of empowering users, has to be balanced against its disadvantages and judgements made in relation to particular health problems. For diseases such as cancer that require complex medical interventions, large institutions have the advantages of specialized facilities and expertise. For chronic health problems, non-institutional care can place intolerable burdens on informal carers.

The third characteristic associated with community health care is the attempt to utilize community resources, primarily within the family (Strauss and Corbin, 1988; Dalley, 1988). The cynical interpretation of community care is that it involves making the family responsible for care that previously was provided by the state. The caring community beyond the family is largely a myth in the modern industrialized world (Baldwin, 1993). However, there are wider resources which can be drawn on, including statutory and voluntary agencies and self-help groups, providing that those in need can find their way through the jungle of organizations and services.

The aims of community health care

Community health care aims to promote good health, to prevent ill health and to help people to cope with the consequences of impairment. There is a tension within this definition between the twin aims of prevention and care. Preventative measures, e.g. genetic screening, may be interpreted as implicitly devaluing those among whom prevention has failed. Abberley (1987) discusses this potential conflict, in an exploration of disability as an oppressive social label. 'What is required is essentially an attitude of ambivalence towards impairment.... The key distinction that must be made is between the prevention of impairment on the one hand, and attitudes to and treatment of people who are already impaired on the other' (p. 9).

Achievement of these aims requires forms of support over and above those given by statutory health agencies, including those provided by government (e.g. promoting full employment), social work and educational services, welfare, housing and voluntary agencies, self-help groups and informal carers. It includes support given to informal carers as well as to those with health problems.

WHAT ARE PERSPECTIVES?

The final conceptual issue to be discussed in this chapter is the nature of perspectives. A perspective is a way of understanding a situation through locating it within a personal frame of reference. A full analysis of perspectives would require consideration of a range of psychological and sociological topics, including perception, cognition, memory, language, communication, attitudes, attribution, negotiation and social influence. The present brief discussion will be confined to three general points: firstly, that perspectives need to be understood at multiple levels; secondly, that a person's perspective includes his/her views of others' perspectives; and thirdly, that perspectives are not fully open to conscious awareness.

Levels of perspective

Perspectives can be thought of as existing at multiple levels, ranging from core, bedrock assumptions – e.g. about the nature of health problems – through to opinions about details – e.g. about specific aspects of care. At deeper levels, perspectives are more general, and can be applied to a wider range of phenomena, but are vaguer in detail, e.g. 'I have faith in modern medicine'. At shallower levels, a perspective is more specific, but its range of convenience is narrower, e.g. 'I am happy to have my baby in hospital because my doctor says it is safer'.

The meaning of the detail of individual perspectives will often be lost unless it is related to broader presuppositions which are easier to overlook. For example, Clarke, in Chapter 8, describes the resistance of some informal carers to respite care for relatives suffering from dementia. Wellmeaning health professionals saw respite care as giving informal carers a much needed break. But for informal carers it could represent a devastating admission that their relationship with the dementing person was no longer normal.

The spiral of perspectives

Our perspectives on situations involving other people include perceptions, correct or incorrect, of how they view the situation. These perspectives on perspectives have been called **meta-perspectives** (Laing, Phillipson and Lee, 1966). For example, users of community health services will usually have views, accurate or not, about how they are seen by health service providers. Some of the adults with learning difficulties discussed in Chapter 10, for instance, felt that staff at their adult training centres regarded them as children and underestimated their abilities.

Higher levels of perspective are possible, limited only by cognitive complexity. For example, a meta-meta-perspective is a perspective on a meta-perspective. However, we will not go any further up the spiral of perspectives!

Perspectives and meta-perspectives can also be considered across interpersonal relationships, in terms of correspondences between various levels. In the above example, formal carers at adult training centres reported that they felt that adults were not achieving their full potential, mainly because their parents held them back. There was thus a gap between formal carers' expressed perspectives on adults' capabilities and the meta-perspectives of adults who thought that formal carers saw them as children.

User perspectives are complex and we need to consider not only how users see carers but how they think that carers see them.

Consciousness and perspectives

Most psychologists, not only Freudians, would accept a distinction between 'mental' and 'conscious'. Some of what a person knows can be inferred from their behaviour by an observer, but the person cannot necessarily bring this knowledge into conscious awareness. For example, young children demonstrate a good grasp of the grammar of their native language in speech but are quite incapable of describing the complex system of rules that they have learnt.

It cannot be assumed that people necessarily 'know their own minds' and are therefore fully capable of describing their perspectives to researchers. However, for the purposes of this book, we will follow Kelly's (1955) famous dictum, quoted slightly out of context. 'If you don't know what's wrong with a client, ask him; he may tell you!' (p. 140).

The source material for the book is what users can tell us about their perspectives in response to questions obtained through research techniques which include participant observation, focus groups, interviews and questionnaires.

CONCLUSION

This chapter has focused on definitional issues. The main argument has been that terms like 'market', 'user', 'community', 'health' and 'care' need to be considered as elements in language games. The idea of a 'market' originally described a social mechanism which gives end consumers direct purchasing power, but has been applied to an arrangement, admittedly qualified as 'internal', that does not do so. The concept of 'community' has been extended from the traditional idea of structural community to describe, for example, residents of a locality within a conurbation. 'Health', in the broad sense in which it is used today, seems to describe states which are consistent with the observer's values, e.g. conformity to social norms. 'Care' is used to describe activities which may be practical and/or emotional, paid or unpaid, institutionally or domestically located.

Language games allow terms to be used flexibly in a variety of contexts. The price paid is increased risk that differences between phenomena described by the same label will be overlooked. Improved understanding of user perspectives, the topic introduced in the next chapter, can help to restore value to over-exploited terms by grounding them in users' own concerns and experiences.

Utilitarian, historical and methodological issues

Bob Heyman

That night in my quiet study room I thought about the difficult problem. How could I teach this blind child? I had no idea. After a while it suddenly occurred to me that first of all I should be in the same condition as a blind person. I rose from my chair and extinguished the light.... In the complete darkness I felt my way around and took violin and bow out of the case and began to play.
SUZUKI, S. (1969) *NURTURED BY LOVE: A NEW APPROACH TO EDUCATION*, P. 57.

INTRODUCTION

Chapter 1 was concerned with the problematic and variable meanings of 'user', 'community', 'health', 'care', 'market' and 'perspective'. Chapter 2 discusses three related topics. Firstly, the potential role of knowledge about user perspectives in improving health care is considered. Secondly, the reasons for the current explosion of interest in user perspectives is explored by means of a brief historical analysis. (A more theoretical analysis of such shifts is provided in Chapter 14, drawing on the ideas of Foucault.) Thirdly, methodological issues associated with researching user perspectives are outlined.

Discussion of the usefulness of researching user perspectives represents something of a 'sales pitch'. Drawbacks and limitations will, however, be owned up to in the critique of consumerism in the second section and the review of methodological problems in the third section of the chapter.

THE VALUE OF LEARNING ABOUT USER PERSPECTIVES

Types of information

Research into user perspectives can cover issues such as:

- concepts of health, illness, disability and handicap;
- knowledge, use, evaluation and perceived integration of available services;
- desired changes in services;
- priorities for the use of scarce resources;
- the needs of people who do not use existing services;
- concealed abuses and malpractices.

Comparing perspectives

The perspectives of people with health problems can be compared with those of formal and informal carers. It has been argued, in Chapter 1, that the nature of their work makes it particularly difficult for paid carers to see health and care through the eyes of users. Gaps between professional and user perspectives are identified in each of the research chapters.

Byrne (Chapter 3) found that accident and emergency patients were most anxious about the social consequences of their condition, but such anxieties were not detected or dealt with by nursing staff, who focused almost entirely on medical problems.

Heyman (Chapter 4) found that the alienated residents of an impoverished housing estate wanted some degree of control over a neighbourhood health centre. The local FHSA, in his view, were not receptive to this idea.

Aarvold and Davies (Chapter 5) found that women receiving antenatal services felt that their need for information was being met only in relation to the physical progress of the birth.

Pearson (Chapter 6) found that gaps developed between the perspectives of new mothers and health visitors as the mothers became more confident and sought more of a partnership. Health visitors sought to retain a primarily monitoring role. Mothers' culturally derived expectancy that babies should be 'naturally' healthy, and the resulting notion of health problems that were not illnesses, conflicted with health visitors' surveillance role.

Davison and Reed (Chapter 7) found that elderly people saw the value of sheltered accommodation mainly in terms of protection from the dangerous world outside. Hostel wardens adopted a medical approach, even though they weren't doctors. The theme of health problems that were not illness reappears at the end of life, since elderly people minimized chronic health problems which, they felt, were a natural consequence of ageing.

Clarke (Chapter 8) identified a conflict between informal carers of the dementing elderly who tried to normalize the problem and formal carers who medicalized it.

Machin and Kingham (Chapter 9) found that people who used disulfiram (a drug which reacts with alcohol to produce intense discomfort) as part of a strategy of flexible drinking felt that they were seen as failures by the medical profession because they did not abstain completely.

Heyman and Huckle (Chapter 10) found gaps between adults with learning difficulties and informal carers, who mostly adopted a 'danger avoidance' approach, and formal carers who wanted the adults to take more risks.

Handyside and Heyman (Chapter 11) concluded that 'mentally ill' people were more likely to define their problems in social than in psychiatric terms, e.g. lack of a job or adequate housing.

Handyside (Chapter 12) found that HIV-positive patients felt that caring professionals needed more experiential 'training' while professionals' own priority was improving their medical knowledge.

Milner and Watson (Chapter 13) found that a support scheme for self-help groups was not a priority for a new district health authority purchaser, even though it was greatly valued by users.

The above research suggests that gaps between provider and user perspectives are common. Endemic misunderstanding, confusion and frustration are the likely consequence. However, researchers may be oversensitive to gaps and misunderstandings such as those summarized above because they make good research material.

Systems of care

Another advantage of learning more about user perspectives is that they can provide holistic pictures of systems of care. Users often receive complex cocktails of health, welfare and social services (see Chapters 8, 11 and 12). People seeking help with health problems must often feel exposed to a bewildering array of services, full of gaps and overlaps, offered by a variety of organizations, with differing philosophies, availability and access. Professionals usually see only parts of such systems, user perceptions of which can often be devastating. For example, four-fifths of a sample of informal carers of elderly and disabled people judged that the community care reforms associated with the NHS and Community Care Act 1990, admittedly in an early stage of implementation, had made no difference to them (Carers' National Association, 1994).

Interfaces between services appear to be a particular weakness in current health services, probably because of the difficulties of coordinating activities of organizations with different cultures and interests. For example, Wiffin (1993) was shocked at the problems she uncovered when she interviewed a small sample of patients discharged after a dynamic hip screw insertion. As a practising nurse, she had previously seen patients only in hospital and had believed that the discharge procedures were effective. In some cases, discharge plans were produced without any discussion with patients. Patients reported a lack of information about possible complications, expected recovery times, medication and visits from other services. One patient who could not climb the stairs to the toilet was having to manage without a commode.

Jones, Lester and West (1994, p. 150) compared older patients' perceptions of information provided at discharge in 1990 and 1992. They concluded that there was as yet no evidence of improvements associated with the implementation of the internal market in health care during this period. For example, 38% of patients reported no discussions with staff before discharge in 1990, and 39% in 1992.

Their own socialization in a particular health discipline makes it harder for health workers to appreciate the perspectives of other professions. Swain (1993) studied members of a 'multidisciplinary' team that included physiotherapists, nurses and teachers in a school for disabled children. He observed that members of each profession felt that their own approach was 'holistic' while that of the other professions was limited by their professional training, nicely illustrating the blinding power of expertise.

Since human beings tend to strive actively to make sense of their worlds, we need to learn how users construct cognitive and evaluative 'maps' of sources of help. The concept of a 'map' suggests that users will impart structure to their experiences, that they will understand the 'cocktail' of services not just as a mixture of isolated elements but as a system with emergent properties.

For older people (Chapter 7), people suffering from dementia and their carers (Chapter 8), adults with learning difficulties (Chapter 10) and HIV-positive people (Chapter 12) one such emergent property can be described in terms of a metaphor of a moving 'escalator' of services. It can be hard to get on or off this escalator, but once on board, the user is carried on, either towards increased dependency and reduced risk or in the opposite direction.

Davison and Reed (Chapter 7) found that older people may take up sheltered accommodation not because they feel unable to live at home but because it improves their perceived access to care which they might need in the future. Once they are 'on the escalator', they are more likely to be offered types of care that minimize risk but increase dependency still further, e.g. residential care.

HIV, like old age, has a probable trajectory of slow decline. Handyside (Chapter 12) describes a patient who lied about his symptoms while he still felt well in order to avoid having to struggle to obtain benefits in the future when his health had deteriorated. In contrast, another patient, close to death, was forced to undergo humiliating rituals to 'prove' his entitlement to a disability allowance.

In the above examples, users joined the care escalator prophylactically in order to pre-empt anticipated future problems. The opposite process is refusing to move towards reduced dependency and greater risk-taking because of anticipated difficulty in regaining safer care, if necessary, in the future. Heyman and Huckle (Chapter 10) found that informal carers of adults with learning difficulties attending adult training centres (ATCs) resisted attempts to move the adults on to more stimulating but also more demanding environments such as sheltered workshops. Their main concern was that the adult would be unable to regain a place in the ATC if he or she was unable to cope outside.

Clarke (Chapter 8), in contrast, suggests that people with dementia and their close relatives may resist getting on to the care escalator because they do not want to acknowledge the downward medical trajectory faced by the dementing person. They may try to normalize the situation for as long as possible by avoiding the diagnostic label of dementia in the early stages of the illness and by resisting health professional efforts to get them to consider the next stage of decline.

The rationality behind the behaviour of users trying to navigate a system of care is often misunderstood by providers who focus on one part of the system. For example, the formal carers interviewed by Heyman and Huckle believed that parents of adults with learning difficulties did not want them to leave ATCs either for psychological reasons (parental over-protectiveness) or for financial reasons (loss of care allowances). People who exaggerate their disabilities in order to obtain state benefits are often portrayed as 'scroungers'. However, for those who anticipate declining health, such behaviour is a rational response to a system that resists legitimate claims for support. Similarly, Clarke found that some formal carers were determined to compel informal carers to face facts and think about the future condition of the dementing person, even against their wishes. But retaining a sense of normality in a relationship with a loved one for as long as possible is a rational response to inevitable, terminal decline.

THE RECENT HISTORY OF IDEAS ABOUT HEALTH CARE

Introduction

During the 1980s, a surge of research interest in user perspectives on community health care began to develop. In Table 2.1 a schema is presented which puts this interest in a wider historical context.

The three models in the schema attempt to describe, in a simplified way, shifts in thinking about health care during the postwar period and to relate these to wider changes in social values.

Table 1.1 Models of health care and the evolution of concern with user perspectives

	Medical model	Social management model	Marketing model
Societal strategic aims	Control of the physical environment	Control of human behaviour	Matching supply and demand
Shortcomings leading to these societal strategic aims	Vulnerability to natural forces	Lack of control of human factors	Value problems and planning failures
Paradigmatic research methodology	Experimental physical research	Experimental social science research	Market research
Characteristic societal interventions	Science and technology	Welfarism	Promotion of mutual adaption between producers and consumers
Health care strategic aims	Cure	Prevention and positive health	Matching needs and provision
Shortcomings leading to these societal strategic aims	Vulnerability to disease	Exclusion of behavioural causes of illness in medical* model	Value problems and vested interests leading to poor outcomes from social management
Characteristic healthcare interventions	Pharmacy; surgery	Health promotion (in practice health education)	Consumerist
Paradigmatic healthcare research methodology	Random controlled trials	Compliance research	User needs and satisfaction research

Although not confined to this country, these changes show up particularly clearly in Britain because of our polarized political system. The beginning of the primacy of the social management model is marked by the foundation of the NHS and the welfare state after the postwar Labour election victory of 1945. 'Social management' will be used as a neutral term to describe an approach which its proponents called 'social democratic', as noted by Goodwin (1990), and its detractors dismissed as 'social engineering' (Szasz, 1970). The rise of the marketing model is associated with the period of Conservative government which began in 1979 and, arguably, peaked with the NHS and Community Care Act 1990.

Each of the three models is analysed below in terms of an underlying strategic aim of 'work' that is dominant in the wider society and that implies a particular way of thinking about health and health care. The paradigm shift to the subsequent model is explained in terms of the emergence of perceived shortcomings in the current model, both in the wider society and in health care. The subsequent model is an attempt to deal with these shortcomings, but is not necessarily 'better' in any absolute sense. An 'empowerment model', whose time has possibly come, is briefly outlined at the end of this section.

Hopefully, the models clarify genuine historical shifts in ways of thinking about health care. But they are, inevitably, over-simplifications. Several ways in which they oversimplify are outlined below.

The three models should be seen as historical accretions. Earlier models that are no longer leading continue to be used. As Nettleton notes in Chapter 14, the 'old guard' manages to survive even after paradigms have moved on. Aarvold and Davies, in Chapter 5, suggest, for example, that child birth services in Britain are currently in a medically dominated time warp. Ironically, the maternally well are being kept in hospital while the sick, e.g. the infirm elderly and those with severe mental illnesses, are being left to the mercies of 'the community'.

Cultural pluralism in views about health care is the norm in complex societies (Unschuld, 1986). Dominant approaches rarely enjoy a monopoly. For example, a powerful public health approach has coexisted with the predominant, reductionist, medical model since the 19th century. But this approach was eclipsed by a more individualized medical model from about the 1870s (Ashton and Seymour, 1988, p. 17).

There is also an element of 'horses for courses', leading to eclecticism, since different models seem appropriate for different kinds of problem. Even the most ardent critic of the medical model would probably welcome it if their appendix was about to burst! Similarly, several areas of the USA have responded to the resurgence of drug-resistant tuberculosis in poor inner-city areas by enforcing compulsory continuation of treatment, a drastic form of social management. More generally, there are certain roles which the state must take responsibility for in a decent society. These include the organization of transfer payments to the sick, the elderly and the unemployed and investment in the human and physical infrastructure.

The progression of ideas about health care can be seen as a succession of discontinuous phases. However, there will usually be periods of transition when one paradigm is giving way to another and quantitative becomes qualitative change. For example, the creation of the welfare state in the 1940s was a revolution which occurred because: 'evolutionary changes in government policy reached a critical mass at which – consciously or unconsciously – they transformed the fundamental nature of the relationship between the state and its citizens' (Lowe, 1993, p. 13).

To make matters even more complicated, models of health care should be seen primarily as ideologies, implicit or explicit, that social actors draw upon to rationalize their actions, as accounting systems. It is not being argued, for example, that Conservative governments since 1979 have refrained from social management, only that its proponents see themselves primarily as creators of 'free markets' that maximize efficiency. The problems with this claim, in the case of the recent 'internal market' in health, have already been discussed, in Chapter 1.

The models of health care are subject to the same double hermeneutic problems as any other social scientific concept. They attempt to describe the frameworks of meaning that health service purchasers, providers and users employ to make sense of health-related interactions. These frameworks are used in language games and are, inevitably, imprecise, variable and overlapping. The systems of meaning that social scientists develop in order to understand social actors' meanings are themselves subject to similar problems, doubling the difficulty.

For example, it is difficult to know whether to classify *The Health of the Nation* (DOH, 1991) as a form of social management, or of marketing. Central government identified five key areas for improvement: coronary heart disease and stroke; cancers; mental illness; HIV/AIDS and sexual health; and accidents. Targets have been set in each of these areas, e.g. to reduce smoking, high levels of alcohol consumption and suicide rates. But the interventions this has given rise to are almost entirely individualistic (Marks, 1994). Major forms of social management needed to achieve the targets, such as measures to reduce poverty, have been ruled out. The government has been unwilling even to take obvious, health-related steps like banning tobacco advertising and sponsorship.

The Health of the Nation could be classified as a form of late decadent social management. It sets societal health targets while excluding social reforms, such as increased taxation of the wealthy, which are needed to achieve these targets but which would conflict with the ideology of the free market. Alternatively, *The Health of the Nation* could be considered as a form of marketing in which the provider specifies a 'product' – targets for health – and then 'sells' them to the public through a campaign designed to change individual behaviour.

Another example of an approach which is not straightforward to classify in terms of the proposed models is the New Public Health. This approach (Ashton and Seymour, 1988, p. 94) advocates large-scale interventions, e.g. concerning unemployment and the environment, in order to empower individuals, simply because it is very difficult for individuals to promote their own health if they have to live in unfavourable conditions. Paradoxically, social management is a necessary means of empowering individuals and families, a point which will be returned to below.

Hybrid, ambiguous and borderline cases, as in the two examples above, are inevitable with any system for classifying complex accounting systems that involve overlapping means and ends.

As a result of historical accretion, pluralism, eclecticism, transitions, problematic ideological claims and classification problems, identification of the leading model at any point in time can never be clear-cut. Hopefully, however, the three models presented in Table 2.1 accurately describe broad shifts in 'the spirit of the times' and provide a context for understanding current interest in user perspectives.

Health care and the wider culture

Ways of thinking that dominate in particular professional groups at specific times have to be compared with ideas prevalent in the wider society. Both similarities and divergences may be expected. Since members of professional groups are also members of the wider society, they are bound to be influenced by the spirit of the time. At the same time, the wider culture is influenced by popularized versions of ideas that originate in the health professions and by the images of themselves which health professionals attempt to promote. Health professionals and the wider public mutually influence each other.

Bowling, Jacobson and Southgate (1993), for example, found that the public prioritized high-technology, life-saving interventions and medical research while GPs and consultants attached greater importance to community services and care for the mentally ill. Thus, at least in a survey, the public adopted a medical model while the doctors adopted a social model.

On the other hand, each professional group has its own traditions, transmitted through socialization processes. These traditions exert a powerful influence on members of a profession, leading to divergences between the professional and the wider culture. For health workers, the world of their profession is likely to loom large in the foreground while 'the community' (i.e. the rest of society) appears small, in the background. One potent source of cultural divergence is the requirement for professionals to come up with solutions to health problems in the here and now, however intractable the problem and however limited their means. For example, GPs appear to have had more faith in the net therapeutic

value of tranquillizers than the general public b
their faith in response to lay beliefs (Gabe and Bu:

Models of health care

The medical model

Scope
Our starting point, much discussed and requiring only a brief mention, is
the medical model, associated with the development of scientific medicine in the latter part of the 19th century. This development was itself
part of a wider growth in the use of science and technology to attempt to
control the physical environment. The medical model defined the aims of
health care in terms of the cure of specific diseases through physical intervention, e.g. drugs, surgery. As a result, wider factors associated with the
development of disease, for example psychological and environmental
factors, were not focused upon.

Persons were reduced to bodies (Chapter 14), and health was implicitly
defined as the absence of disease. This way of thinking legitimized the
power of medical staff, since only they had the 'scientific' expertise necessary to diagnose and treat diseases.

Limitations
By reducing health problems to specific malfunctions of the body, the
medical model fails to take into account social and behavioural processes
associated with the development of diseases, e.g. relationships between
ill-health and social inequality. Nor does the medical model concern itself
with the need to deal with the social and human consequences of
diseases which cannot be cured. As a result, western health systems have
been biased towards high-technology curative medicine and have failed
to make an appropriate response to chronic health problems (Strauss and
Corbin, 1988).

The social management model

Scope
The shortcomings of a purely medical model became more apparent as
mass killer infectious diseases such as smallpox, cholera and typhoid were
largely eliminated in the western world. As life expectancy increased,
management of chronic disease became a more important concern.
Health care now had to deal with the person as well as the body, and the
most appropriate knowledge base was the social rather than the medical
sciences (Chapter 14).

Social management, in health care and other forms of state provision,
was the leading model in Britain in the 30 years following the Second

World War. Social management attempted to promote human welfare through central planning, with the implication, subsequently questioned, that planners know best.

The term 'social management' inevitably covers a family of different labels and approaches (Williams, 1989, Ch. 2) that are beyond the scope of this book. Our main purpose is to analyse the role of user perspectives in health systems. From this perspective, a central feature of social management approaches (e.g. Fabian social democracy in the period after 1945) was their 'technocratic' reliance on social scientific research to determine the optimum means of social management, for example, to relieve poverty or to improve housing. Hence, the issue of power relationships between providers and users of health care was not seen as a central problem. The importance currently given to this issue (Carpenter, 1994) represents a genuine historical transformation in thinking about health and other services.

Two types of method of social management were available. One was to change the structure and fabric of society, e.g. through mass rehousing programmes and the development of the welfare state and the NHS. The second was attempting to change individual behaviour, e.g. through the rapid expansion of social work, the development of family therapy and the use of psychotropic drugs.

Limitations

The knowledge base for the health of persons was not prestigious and apparently robust natural sciences like biomedicine but the methodologically shaky, value-ridden and controversial social sciences. However, health professionals attempted to maintain the same power relationship towards patients, grounded in their 'expert' knowledge as social managers, that they had asserted on the basis of the medical model. The assumptions that the social sciences can be value-free and that the state and its agents act benevolently to maximize public welfare have been widely challenged (Bulmer, 1982; Goodwin, 1990).

The famous and now much criticized WHO (1958) definition of health (part of the founding constitution of 1946) as 'a state of complete physical, mental and social well being, and not merely the absence of disease and infirmity' (p. 459) illustrates the grandiose claims associated with the social management approach to health. The more modest and consumerist WHO (1986) definition of health is discussed in the next part of the chapter.

The main defect in the social management model is that it obscures the need for people, individually and collectively, to make value choices in response to the dilemmas of human existence, for example about the level of risk that they are willing to accept in order to achieve their goals. As one member of the focus groups discussed in Chapter 4 put it: 'Life's about risks. It's because we take risks that we have the quality of life...

You've been in a hospital ward where people have had to stop smoking who were ill, and that might have been their only pleasure, their only comfort.'

Szasz (1970) attacked what he described as a social engineering approach to community health, particularly the claim for a value-free 'science' of mental health. His quotation from the grandly titled Scientific Committee of the World Federation for Mental Health illustrates the approach which he criticized.

> The principles underlying success in attempts to alter cultural conditions in the interests of mental health, and the hazards of such attempts, are very important considerations for practical mental health work... The introduction of changes in a community may be subject to conditions not unlike those which obtain in the case of the child. (Soddy K. (1962) cited in Szasz (1970), p. 38)

The community, in the above quotation, is a child while the mental health worker is, by implication, a parent who can make value choices on its behalf.

Another revealing example of this genre is the work of Skinner (1972), which envisaged a Utopia run by psychologists who would determine the route to human happiness scientifically, a proposition which does not seem to have had much appeal for non-psychologists. The excesses of the social management approach laid it open to attack by the New Right and contributed to the ascendancy during the 1980s of the marketing model. Szasz himself adopted an individualistic, libertarian position (Sedgwick, 1982, Ch. 6), arguing, for example, that state welfare promoted dependency.

By obscuring value dilemmas, the social management model conceals conflicts of interest between providers and users. It assumes that the managers will act benevolently to achieve welfare aims, rather than promoting their own interests. Professional self-definitions promote this lofty ethical stance, but it has aroused considerable scepticism (Hugman, 1992).

The social management model takes for granted the definition of the ends that care should be aiming for, thus obscuring existential dilemmas and conflicts of interest. Unfortunately, the means by which health and welfare are to be achieved have, in practice, been equally problematic. At the societal level, health and welfare systems reproduce racial, sexual and class-based inequalities found in the wider society (Williams, 1989).

Specific interventions designed to improve social conditions or modify individual behaviour in order to promote health have, almost invariably, aroused controversy. Postwar housing estates are being blown up before their time. Economic transfers to the poorest sector of society are alleged to generate a 'dependency culture'. The long-term side effects of tranquillizers, particularly addiction (Tyrer, 1988), may be worse than their supposed benefits, which have themselves been questioned (Goodwin, 1990, p. 11). The side effects of cholesterol-lowering drugs may be worse than the benefits (Hulley *et al.*, 1993). In contrast, moderate alcohol consumption may protect against heart disease (Peele, 1993) and cannabis may have medicinal properties (Munro, Thomas and Abu Shaar, 1993). Even smoking has partial defenders who see it as a necessary support for people who live in difficult conditions. Doubt and controversy, justified or not, have weakened the credibility of health and other 'experts' and, paradoxically, empowered people who demand to make their own choices (Giddens, 1991).

Because the ends are controversial and the means dubious, people have not fully complied with health professional advice and have made their own minds up about which parts of the advice to follow. For example, there is still widespread prejudice against HIV sufferers (Macdonald and Smith, 1990), despite frequent media campaigns to demystify the disease. At the same time, the impact of 'safe sex' campaigns on the young heterosexual population appears to have been negligible (Macdonald and Smith, 1990), perhaps because young people consider the current low levels of personal risk worth taking. Macdonald and Smith's (1990) recommendation of 'a coherent and coordinated health education programme which tackles attitudes surrounding prejudice and complacency as a first step' (p. 67) illustrates their faith in a social management response to low compliance.

Since people fail to fully follow advice designed to promote their health, welfare and happiness, then research into compliance may be resorted to in an attempt to make social management more effective. As shown in Table 2.1, compliance research supports the social management model in the same way that biomedical research supports the medical model and consumer needs and satisfaction research underpin the marketing model.

Thousands of studies of compliance have been carried out since the 1960s, and the Medline database records over 1000 studies worldwide between 1990 and the first half of 1993. The main conclusion (Becker, 1974) has been that patients will only comply if the treatment fits in with their own health beliefs and wants! Much compliance research is based on the implicit assumption, central to the social management model, that people who do not comply are doing something wrong (Trostle, 1988).

An alternative to seemingly ineffective psychological methods of attempting to increase compliance is the technical fix which aims to deprive people of choice through the use of sophisticated technology. For example, it seems easier to fly helicopters over inner-city localities or to deploy video cameras in town centres than to tackle the causes of crime. Other instances of the technical fix approach to social management in health care are given below.

Remote sensors to monitor the health of the population are being developed in Japan (Hodgson, 1992). Already in production to detect diabetes in residents of old peoples' homes, these sensors are placed in toilets and, it is envisaged, will eventually monitor signs of a variety of diseases including cancer, infections and gut functions. The initiators have suggested that the sensors could be connected to doctors' offices, providing automatic detection and long-term monitoring of disease.

An example which is closer to home is the use of electronic tagging to control the movements of elderly people in residential care, particularly in NHS hospitals (Counsel and Care, 1993).

Disulfiram may be considered a technical fix for drinking problems, since users experience unpleasant side effects if they attempt to consume alcohol. Machin and Kingham's research, in Chapter 9, shows that users frequently adapt disulfiram to their own ends, e.g. to give themselves control over drinking bouts, and that successful use of the drug requires a wider pattern of change, for example finding alternative ways of structuring time meaningfully. Disulfiram in isolation appears to be an ineffective technical fix for problem drinking.

Technical fixes either violate human rights, are easily circumvented, or both.

The marketing model

Scope

During the 1980s, New Right governments, particularly in Britain and the USA, reacted against the social management approach to health and welfare, driven by neoliberal philosophy (e.g. Friedman, 1962), and aided, as noted above, by the excesses and failures of social management. The neoliberal position asserts that economic development and welfare can best be achieved through the promotion of 'free markets' that allow individuals to act in their own interests with a minimum of state interference.

State intervention to promote health and welfare is viewed as problematic, from the neoliberal perspective, for three reasons. Firstly, it is seen as promoting a 'dependency culture'. Secondly, it is seen as a drain on public expenditure, leading to increased taxation and reduced individual freedom to spend disposable income. Thirdly, it is seen as giving providers monopoly power, unconstrained by 'market discipline', which they will exploit. Providers, from the framework of a marketing model, do not know best. They inevitably put their interests over those of the people they are supposed to serve if their power is unchecked.

Cynicism about the motivation and efficiency of providers has been one of the main ideological forces behind the reforms associated with the 1990 NHS and Community Care Act, although it is inevitably confounded with the drive to reduce public expenditure and combat the alleged dependency culture. The wider manifestations of this cynicism, in the actions of Conservative governments during the 1980s, have included curtailment of the autonomy of local authorities, privatization, Citizen's Charters and the imposition of 'performance indicators', regardless of their dubious validity, e.g. league tables for schools.

The marketing model attempts to give power over decision-making to those who purchase goods and services directly or through taxation. Taken at face value, the consumer is 'king' and determines the goods and services that will be produced, via purchasing decisions.

Wider socioeconomic changes have supported the shift towards a marketing model of care. Rapid increases in the proportion of elderly people in western societies, combined with lower rates of economic growth as the world centre for manufacturing moves to South-East Asia, have created a crisis in the financing of the welfare state. In Britain, this crisis has been accentuated, since 1979, by reductions in taxation for the wealthy and the New Right political imperative, as yet unrealized, to reduce the overall burden of taxation.

At the same time, a wider consumerism has developed, reflecting rising expectations among the economically active section of the population, who have experienced ever increasing affluence in the postwar period. The parallel shift towards consumerism in health care (Griffiths, 1988a) is associated with more critical attitudes towards health care, and conflicts with the traditional ethos of the NHS in its restriction of choice, use of rationing and producer power.

The WHO (1986) definition of health, which should be compared with the earlier one discussed above, illustrates the transformation which is taking place. Health is defined in terms of 'the extent to which an individual or group is able, on the one hand, to realize aspirations and satisfy needs; and, on the other hand, to change or cope with the environment. Health is, therefore, seen as a resource for everyday life, not the objective of living' (p. 73).

Health, in the above quotation, is seen as relative to the aspirations of individuals or groups, and so can only be defined in relation to user perspectives.

However, health systems have to meet the needs of populations, not individuals. The 'market' must be segmented into sections likely to have different needs, for example using a life-cycle approach. The needs of each segment must be identified, through user-perspective research. Pickin and St Leger (1993) address their book to 'those who seek to assess the health needs of populations in a systematic manner. Matching resources for health, in particular services, to needs is the core task of health services policy' (p. v).

Limitations

There is no reason to suppose that the marketing model will be any more permanent, as the leading model, than have been the medical or the social management model. Three related weaknesses can be suggested. Firstly, consumer satisfaction can be achieved through any mix of changing services in the direction that consumers want and persuading them to want what it is convenient and profitable to provide. Given the power and prestige of providers such as the medical profession and drug companies, it is probable that people will be persuaded to 'want' dubious remedies, e.g. cosmetic breast implants for women, cholesterol-lowering drugs.

More generally, consumers are allowed choice only over peripheral features of goods and services. In Chapter 14, Nettleton, drawing on the work of Castel (1991), describes the present phase as one in which populations are managed according to epidemiological risk factors, personal relationships between users and health professionals are weakened and groups who do not participate in postindustrial society are marginalized. This vision is much less benign than that of Pickin and St Leger (1993). It suggests a system which processes people rather than one which adapts to individual needs.

Secondly, consumerist strategies which focus on individuals provide no means of meeting collective needs, with potentially disastrous consequences. For example, individual parents may rationally decide not to immunize their children, in order to avoid the risk of brain damage. But, if all parents were to adopt this strategy, the health consequences would be catastrophic. Similarly, the rise in crime and civil disorder in inner cities is linked to our failure to deal with social problems like poverty and unemployment (Benyon, 1993).

Thirdly, giving individuals choice over collectively funded services can lead to escalating costs, at least in 'market' systems in which providers have a direct interest in 'selling' as much care as possible. This is, undoubtedly, one of the reasons why British 'consumers' have not been given control over health and community services, as discussed in Chapter 1. For example, in December 1992, the Social Services Inspectorate issued an official guideline stating that individual care plans, now required for disabled people, should not record user preferences where these could not be met for financial reasons. GP fundholders and district health authorities have a similar rationing function.

It is instructive to compare 'consumerism' in British health care with that in France. Health care in France (Mermet, 1993) is mainly funded through a national insurance scheme which covers 75% of the cost of care and is intended to be universal. More than 75% of the population have additional insurance covering the entire cost of care and this group consumes more *per capita* health care than those who have to meet part of the cost.

Patients can consult as many doctors as they want, or refer themselves directly to a specialist or hospital of their choice, and can readily obtain diagnostic tests. At least one-third of patients ask for a second opinion. Payments to doctors are based on referrals, thus giving patients real consumer power. French visitors express shock at the lack of choice, shortages, waiting lists and drabness which they see in the British NHS. However, the French spend a higher proportion of their national wealth on health care than do the British (*L'État de la France*, 1992), and are the largest *per capita* consumers of medicines in the world.

The USA private insurance system has encountered similar problems, since insured users do not purchase health care individually and have little incentive to curtail costs. This system combines poor cost control with lack of universality and is ripe for reform.

British users of the state system do not have direct purchasing power, as they do in France. The agents who are supposed to take decisions on their behalf can only treat them as consumers if they can discover what users want. This is one reason for the current concern with investigating user perspectives (Pickin and St Leger, 1993). For this version of consumerism to 'work', it has to be assumed that purchasers and/or providers, having identified user wishes, will benevolently translate them into practice. Scepticism about this assumption has already been expressed in Chapter 1, in the discussion of the new 'internal market' for health.

Consumerism has reached an impasse, itself part of a more general crisis, as the ecological costs of more and more economic growth and the costs to communities of the globalization of production begin, increasingly, to outweigh the benefits (Beck, 1992). City dwellers, for example, cannot 'buy' clean air, and are faced with ever-increasing risks of asthma and cancer from car pollutants, as traffic density is allowed to increase remorselessly.

It is theoretically possible to envisage a health care market in which the behaviour of providers would be constrained by consumers, through their decisions about how to spend limited resources. Such a system could operate if consumers were left to individually purchase health care from competing suppliers, or given a limited number of vouchers by the state for this purpose. Individual consumers would be motivated to use their limited resources as efficiently as possible, to purchase the health care which they themselves selected.

Because of the complexity of health care decisions, consumers would, in this imaginary system, be at the mercy of commercial interests marketing their products. (The recent fiasco in Britain involving large numbers of people being sold inappropriate pensions illustrates what can happen when sellers of complex products are allowed to prey on the public.) In this imaginary market system, people who ran out of money or vouchers would simply be denied care or would receive poor-quality care from safety-net providers.

Given that individual needs for health care vary so greatly, it might be possible to give consumers different amounts of vouchers, depending upon their medical condition and social circumstances. However, it is difficult to see how allocation could be anything other than a bureaucratic nightmare which would make the present inequities between fundholding and non-fundholding GPs pale into insignificance. And consumers who 'wasted' their vouchers, perhaps under commercial pressure, would be deprived of further care. (Vouchers for specific purposes, for example to provide a more flexible alternative to concessionary bus fares (Le Grand and Bartlett, 1993, p. 9), are not being criticized. What is under attack is the idea of a system of health and social care based primarily on vouchers.)

Health systems cannot both be designed to protect individuals and be made efficient through market discipline. Neither the American system (consumer cartels buying private insurance) nor the French system (reimbursement by the state) nor the current British system (proxy purchasing 'on behalf of' users) creates a system in which end users constrain providers to act efficiently by making individual decisions about how to use their own scarce resources.

It is time to stop developing variants of quasi-markets of care and to consider alternatives which do not involve reverting back to producer monopolies.

Empowerment: the next model?

The much discussed concept of empowerment (e.g. Kilian, 1988) often evokes cynicism, understandable in response to the mushrooming of 'empowerment groups' in trusts and even the NHSME. However, the promotion of genuine user empowerment may be a way of progressing beyond the impasse of consumerism and is particularly appropriate with wicked problems, which cannot have correct solutions.

The model focuses on commonalities and differences of perspective and interest, both within and between various groups of 'stakeholders' in health systems: actual users; the wider public; health workers and their collective representatives, such as trade unions; and national and local government. The concept of 'interest' is itself problematic (Lukes, 1974; Means and Smith, 1994, pp. 71–2). As noted in the discussion of symbolic interaction in Chapter 1, interactants may attempt to respond to potential conflicts of interest by attempting to influence others' definitions of their own interests and definitional power is not equally distributed. However, an empowerment model based on user perspectives requires the assumption that, in appropriately facilitating conditions, individuals can validly articulate their own interests.

Management of differences of perspective and interest requires the development of power-sharing mechanisms. For example, 'free market' approaches to paid health workers, which treat them as an expendable resource in competitive struggles, simply disaffect the work force and so are self-defeating. (They also create stress-related health problems.) The empowerment model would treat paid health workers as stakeholders, without whose support an efficient, high-quality health service is impossible. But this model, in contrast to the social management model, would also point up systematic differences in perspective and interest between providers and users of health services. Both market jungles and worker paradises need to be avoided.

In the empowerment model, the sharp distinction which the marketing model makes between users, producers and purchasers of health care is abandoned. Users are seen as the primary producers of their own health (Stacey, 1976) and as having rights and obligations, as citizens to participate in decisions about the provision of care. The growth of self-help, advocacy and disability rights groups since the 1970s suggests that users are seeking to be more than consumers, and to contribute to the provision of services. This growth can itself be seen as part of a wider development of 'new social movements' involving green, ethnic minority, women's and gay movements as well as more local community and tenants' associations (Mayo, 1994, p. 58).

As Mayo argues, these movements have an important part to play in enabling people to participate directly in the management of society and so empowering them. But they cannot be a substitute for collective democratic control. The new social movements tend to be unevenly distributed, fragmented and schismatic. They may either be transitory or become institutionalized, as they make compromises with existing power structures in order to survive.

The most important way of empowering people to maintain their own health is external to the health care system and beyond the scope of this book. It is to tackle relative and absolute poverty, since health problems are unduly concentrated among the poor (Davey Smith, Bartley and Blane, 1990), and poverty deprives people of choices. The incomes of the bottom 10% of the population dropped substantially between 1979 and 1991 (HMSO, 1993) in a period of generally rising prosperity, a shameful trend.

The wicked problem is that individuals and families, particularly the disadvantaged, can only be empowered if people in general give up some of their individual freedom to the state, e.g. by accepting fair taxes for the better off and public borrowing for environmentally friendly investments that reduce structural unemployment.

The power of the state should be checked through improved democratic control, not through reducing its functions to a minimum. The New Right solution of cutting down the state as far as possible is merely creating a mass of people who are unable to help themselves because they are impoverished and unhealthy, like the residents of the housing estate discussed in Chapter 4. A Back to Basics campaign is needed to reassert our collective obligation to support the sick, the elderly and the structurally unemployed, particularly families with children.

The 'democratic deficit' caused by increased centralization and the growth of quangos needs to be reversed. Elected regional governments could adapt national policy to local needs and culture and consider regional health in its wider context (employment, poverty, housing, the environment, leisure, education). Regional governments should be responsible for services that require strategic planning, including, in the health field, specialist medical care (e.g. cancer treatment centres of excellence), environmental and public health, research and health professional education.

Elected regional governments would provide indirect democratic control over the formal health system. The well-known, but controversial, Oregon experiment in priority setting (Dixon and Welch, 1991) illustrates the way in which the public can influence resource allocation in a regional health system more directly through expressing their own preferences in surveys and public meetings.

Local authorities should become democratically accountable commissioners of health and social services. Ironically, in community health services such as midwifery, health promotion, health visiting and district nursing, this reform would involve a move back to the situation which existed before the Local Government Act of 1974 transferred control to health authorities. Chaper 5 argues that this change exacerbated the over-medicalization of birth.

An organizational model for the local provision of user-friendly services which has, as its starting point, residents' interrelated health, social, environmental and economic needs, rather than organizational divisions, is needed. Wistow (1994) discusses a variety of models, including unified 'health' and 'social' commissioning by local authorities (p. 35). However, organizational unification should not be equated with integration of services. For example, existing local authority social services, housing, leisure, environmental and education departments appear to coexist quite independently. Integrated locality planning, with direct resident representation and participation, is one possible means of bridging organizational schisms, and giving local people a sense of ownership of 'their' services (see the last part of Chapter 4).

At the level of specific service provision, a variety of measures that empower users and potential users should be considered. Community health councils could take regulatory, rather than consultative powers. Users (e.g. people with disabilities and their carers) and front-line workers could be significantly represented on the governing bodies of providers. The dilemma of representativeness versus activism will have to be confronted, since activists are needed to operate a participatory health system but do not necessarily represent the views of fellow citizens.

Local authority commissioners should direct resources into supporting and evaluating the activities of self-help and community groups (Chapter 13). Such groups are particularly appropriate for the sorts of long-term conditions that community health care mainly deals with, because they start from members' concerns, empower them to tackle their own problems, draw upon lived experience rather than scientific knowledge and create genuine communities.

Increased financial support for self-help groups is a significant potential benefit arising from the NHS and Community Care Act of 1990. However, such groups should be seen as complementing state provision, not replacing it. As already noted, they tend to be impermanent, fragmented and unevenly distributed. Above all, as argued in Chapter 13, they need systematic support from statutory services. Power relationships between self-help groups and statutory services will, inevitably, be problematic and forms of power-sharing need to be developed.

At an individual level, ways need to be found to give users of health services more direct power over the care that they receive. The contrast between the British internal market and power given to French patients to choose their own treatment could not be sharper. Ways of giving users direct choices that do not lead to uncontrollable escalation of costs and unnecessary medicalization need to be found.

METHODOLOGICAL ISSUES

Introduction

Research into user perspectives cannot begin to be useful unless the findings fully, accurately and sensitively reflect their beliefs, feelings and aspirations. The present discussion does no more than highlight major issues associated with the research chapters which follow.

A fully adequate methodology for investigating user perspectives on community health care requires that the right people are asked the right questions, that they answer in ways which reflect their true beliefs and feelings and that their answers are interpreted correctly.

Getting the 'right' people

Getting the 'right' people requires that the researcher defines the population of theoretical interest, identifies its members, gains access to them and persuades them to participate in the research. Each of these requirements is theoretically and/or practically problematic.

Defining the population

Even defining the boundaries of the population can be troublesome. Difficulty arises where the definition of the health problem is conceptually confused, as in the case of mental illness (Chapter 11), or when classification of milder cases is marginal, as with low-level disability associated with old age (Chapter 7), mild dementia (Chapter 8) and learning difficulties (Chapter 10).

When it is difficult to define the boundaries of a human population, it is tempting to fall back on social labelling. Individuals will be included in the population if they define themselves, or are defined, as belonging to a particular category, usually through the receipt of services.

Inclusion in the research population will then depend upon the vagaries of service provision and self-selection by service users. The view of community health services which emerges from such research will exclude potential users who were not offered access to services or who chose not to use them. This limitation is apparent in most of the research chapters in this book, since samples were largely obtained through service contacts.

Gatekeeping

Accurate and up-to-date lists of service users are unlikely to be available and users must be accessed through 'gatekeeper' service providers. Gatekeeping problems are discussed by most contributors to this volume, a reflection of their importance in research practice.

The problem is not so much that some organizations refuse to open the gate, but that these are likely to be ones that fear that they will get a 'bad press'. The poorer organizations, from a user perspective, will be excluded from the research and the results will be unduly positive. This happened with the GP practices discussed in Chapter 4.

The aims of sampling

Within the classic quantitative approach, e.g. user satisfaction surveys, the researcher aims to obtain as representative a sample as possible, ideally by inviting a probability sample to participate, and (hopefully) obtaining a high response rate.

In qualitative research, the investigator may still seek to obtain a representative sample so as to explore typical cases (e.g. Chapter 6). However, Patton (1990) has identified 15 other aims for qualitative sampling. For example, 'maximum variation' sampling looks for commonalities and differences across conditions which vary as much as possible. Theoretical sampling is 'sampling on the basis of concepts that have proven theoretical relevance to the evolving theory' (Strauss and Corbin, 1990, p. 176), and takes place through repeated cycles of sampling, data collection and analysis.

In practice, qualitative and quantitative methods are often combined (Bryman, 1988) in a variety of ways. One of the most important is the development of simple counts (Silverman, 1985) and even measures of relationship, based on the coding of qualitative data (Chapter 10). Once the qualitative researcher becomes concerned with counts, considerations of representativeness become relevant and there is a tension between this concern and the aim of maximum variability. If the research is done in several stages it may be possible to sample maximum variations in the early stages, and then to look for representative samples of 'typical variations' later on.

Recruiting users

Once through the gates the researcher must, for ethical reasons, explicitly ask individual users to agree to participate and must emphasize that refusal will not in any way affect the services they receive.

The lower the response rate, the more the sample is self-selecting and the greater the danger that it will not be representative. For example, evidence will be presented in Chapter 4 that participation in a survey of patient satisfaction with GPs was lower among the young and those from lower socioeconomic groups. These groups were probably least satisfied with their GPs.

In general, the questionnaire surveys in this book had lower response rates than those involving interviews. The postal survey of patient satisfaction with GPs (Chapter 4) yielded a response rate of 79%, but only after non-respondents had been sent two additional invitations to participate. The initial response rate was only 46%. It is comparable to the rate of 51%, reported in Chapter 13, for a survey of members of self-help groups although in this study some groups had previously declined to participate. The questionnaires given to women attending maternity units in a socially deprived area (Chapter 5) were returned by only 28%. However, there is evidence from the GP patient survey and other research (e.g. Harrington *et al.*, 1993) that younger people and those from lower socioeconomic classes have lower response rates generally. The 28% response rate in this study may be comparable with those found in the studies mentioned above.

In sharp contrast, a health needs survey carried out by members of a community group in a deprived area (Chapter 4) achieved a response rate of only 2%, probably because it was initiated by lay people who lacked credibility. This situation is ironic because, as Chapter 4 will try to show, 'emancipatory research' initiated by the researched themselves may be a more effective way of enabling people to articulate their own agendas than research which is controlled by professionals or academics (Zarb, 1992).

Most of the samples discussed in this volume were obtained through personal requests to be interviewed rather than anonymized surveys. Response rates were generally higher, 75% or above. Rates of around 100% were obtained for elderly people living alone in sheltered accommodation, but not those living with a partner (Chapter 9), adults with learning difficulties (Chapter 10) and the mentally ill (Chapter 11). Social isolation, perhaps, motivated members of these groups to talk to an interviewer. Similarly, the 100% participation rate obtained among patients in accident and emergency departments (Chapter 3) may be explained in part by their boredom and anxiety.

A lower response rate, 48%, was obtained in a study of informal carers of the dementing elderly (Chapter 8), with the lowest rate among male carers. Problems were experienced in recruiting any HIV-positive people in an area of low prevalence (Chapter 12). However, the sample had to be obtained indirectly, through formal carers, in order to preserve anonymity and it is unclear how far the difficulty arose with these 'gate-keepers' rather than with respondents. Handyside notes that recruitment in an area of high prevalence was much easier. Members of the target populations in both these studies may have been reluctant to participate because they had only recently become members of stigmatized groups (carers of the demented and HIV-positive people).

The attitudes of potential respondents to participating in research have to be understood within their own frames of reference. For example, Davison and Reed (Chapter 7) found that all the residents of sheltered accommodation living alone, but none of the married couples, were willing to be interviewed. The married couples said that they felt healthy, and, therefore, did not think that their participation was relevant. In fact, the researchers would have been particularly interested in finding out why these couples were in sheltered accommodation.

Asking the 'right' questions

Provider- and user-oriented questions

It is easy for the researcher to ask questions that are directed at provider rather than user concerns (McIver, 1993, p. 3). For example, the researcher may be interested in perceptions of a specific profession while users are concerned with their health problems. Quantitative research, because it is structured and preplanned, is perhaps more likely than qualitative research to overlook user concerns.

For example, an important topic in the GP-initiated survey discussed in Chapter 4 was user perceptions of the waiting and consulting rooms. However, this topic was not mentioned once by members of focus groups who could direct discussion towards their own concerns. The condition of their waiting and consulting rooms may be more important to GPs, who see them daily, than to patients.

Initial qualitative exploratory work can help the researcher to direct the focus of quantitative questions towards user concerns.

The meaning of the questions

Unless researcher and respondent have a similar interpretation of the meaning of the questions, misunderstanding is inevitable. Belson (1981) concluded from intensive qualitative follow-up that misunderstanding was common even for simple standardized questions such as 'What do you usually do when the television advertisements come on?'. For example, 'you' was often interpreted to include other members of the respondent's family, and 'usually' had varying interpretations.

The problems with question wording seemed to Belson to be quite intractable. 'Good' questions generated as many problems as those which had deliberate design faults, e.g. 'double-barrelled' questions with two questions rolled into one. Such problems are inherent in 'language games', discussed in Chapter 1, because meanings in natural language are flexible, and so fuzzy.

Asking the 'right' questions is much harder for researchers investigating user perspectives on community health care than it was for Belson, who deliberately chose 'easy' topics. Community health care is associated with issues concerning sickness, disability, dependency and death, and so is inevitably emotionally charged. And differences in the backgrounds, experiences and perspectives of researchers and respondents are likely to be particularly wide. Again, qualitative research, at least in the initial stages of the investigation, may help to reduce misunderstanding by promoting feedback and allowing respondents to reply in their own terms.

Obtaining valid answers

If the respondent has understood the question in the way intended, valid data will only be obtained if the answer reflects his or her perspective. Users may not necessarily have 'a' perspective, because the topic is of little concern to them or because their views are variable, depending upon specific experiences. Respondents may come up with an answer simply to satisfy the researcher.

Even if the user is able to articulate a perspective, he or she may or may not be willing to reveal personal information or criticize services. The social context in which questioning takes place is as important a determinant of answers as the questions themselves.

The social context includes the setting in which the questions are asked (e.g. home versus an institution), the perceived role of the researcher (e.g. membership of a provider profession under evaluation) and the personal relationship between researcher and researched. Developing and maintaining trust through an ongoing relationship is usually a prerequisite for gaining information in highly sensitive areas.

Anthropologists and sociologists use participant observation to investigate the perspectives of special groups from the inside, particularly where there are barriers against outsiders. Researchers can investigate client perspectives while in a provider or observer role (Chapter 3), and may obtain invaluable 'inside' information. They cannot participate as users unless the researcher belongs to the group whose needs are being investigated or pretends to be a member of this group (Rosenhan, 1973), an ethically dubious procedure.

Interpreting the answers

Quantitative and qualitative data

Although quantitative and qualitative methods are considered separately below, the distinction between them is not clear-cut. They can be combined in various ways (Bryman, 1988), as already noted in the discussion of sampling. For example, qualitative can be converted to quantitative data through coding (Chapter 10). Or, as in Chapter 13, quotations from 'open' questions can be used to illustrate descriptive statistics derived from 'closed' questions which allow only a limited number of responses so as to permit quantification.

The last part of Chapter 11 shows how quantitative data can be used to select and organize qualitative data. In this case, clients' accounts of their mental health problems were related to positive and negative changes in a quantitative measure of self-reported mental health. Clients who had changed positively on the mental health questionnaire appeared to have also shifted from psychological to more social situational accounts of their problems.

Analysing quantitative data

Quantitative data can be used to generate descriptions of single variables and analysis of relationships between variables. Both are subject to limitations.

Descriptive information about user perspectives usually covers use and evaluation of services and may be specific or global. An inherent limitation of using surveys to evaluate services is that results depend upon the format of questions (Fitzpatrick and Hopkins, 1983). They may tell us more about question wording than about perceptions of the service. It is easy to code responses to closed questions reliably, but their validity is problematic.

Relational information can be of two kinds. Firstly, variants of a service can be compared using standard questions. For example, Mangen and Griffith (1982) compared patient perspectives on treatment by psychiatrists *versus* community psychiatric nurses and showed that patients preferred the latter. An important feature of the study was random allocation to the two treatment groups, ensuring that overall they were likely to be roughly comparable before the treatments commenced.

Studies of different variants of a service are perhaps more useful than simple descriptive studies because they allow comparisons with the methodology held constant. Chapters 5 and 11 discuss quasi-experimental comparisons of community-oriented and more conventional interventions in the fields of midwifery and mental health. Chapter 4 describes a comparison of user perceptions of different GP practices using a standard postal questionnaire. GPs were able to use the results to see how they 'scored' compared with other practices in their county.

However, it is not usually possible to randomly allocate users to variants of the service that are likely to have different mixes of users, e.g. in terms of age, social class and ethnicity. As a result, differences in the popularity of variants of a service may reflect differences in clientele rather than the quality of provision.

It is possible, in the absence of random allocation, to control statistically for factors that might be associated with user perspectives (Chapter 4), or to match users receiving different variants of a service on such factors (Chapters 5 and 11). But it can never be certain that control or matching is complete because it is always possible that the researchers have failed to match on other relevant but unknown variables (Cook and Campbell, 1979). For example, the initial samples of mentally ill people discussed in Chapter 11 were not matched for living in a hostel. An additional sample had to be recruited after differences between the experimental and control groups were discovered.

In many cases, users will select, or be referred to, a particular service because of their attitudes, making comparisons with the control group problematic. In the research discussed in Chapter 11, clients with mental health problems using a voluntary agency were less satisfied with their CPNs, and had had less frequent contacts with formal services, than a matched control group. They appear to have chosen the voluntary agency because they felt that statutory services were not meeting their needs.

Experimental community interventions can usually only be tried out on a small scale, and this may limit their effectiveness. For example, Aarvold and Davies point out in Chapter 5 that it has not as yet been possible to try out a home-based midwifery service for an entire community in Britain. It is difficult to compare home with hospital births, because women who give birth at home are self-selecting and may often have to work against the grain of local provision, e.g. against medical opposition.

User demographic, psychological or other characteristics can themselves be related to user perspectives in order to try to explain why user perceptions of similar services differ (Chapter 4).

There are two major problems with interpreting results from this kind of research. Firstly, relationships between demographic variables and user satisfaction tend to be very weak, even if statistically significant, and are often inconsistent. For example, relationships between socioeconomic status and satisfaction with GPs, never strong, vary from study to study, and this inconsistency itself requires explanation (Fox and Storms, 1981).

The second problem is that statistical relationships are not necessarily causal. In survey research, it is always possible that the relationship between two variables, A and B, arises not because A causes B, but because B causes A or because another variable, C, causes both A and B. Statistical controls, as in Chapter 4, can be used to eliminate the possible influence of known 'confounding' variables (Marsh, 1982, p. 76). But they cannot be used to exclude the possible influence of unknown variables. This is particularly worrying when, as in much survey research, relationships between variables are weak.

It is not being argued that such research into relationships between user satisfaction and demographic factors is useless, only that it has limitations. It may be worth knowing, for example, that younger people are less satisfied with a service, even if the relationship is weak and difficult to interpret. Novice researchers are advised to avoid the temptation to do this kind of research just because it is relatively easy to obtain demographic and psychological test data, or because quantitative research seems more 'scientific'.

Analysing qualitative data

The reader is referred to Dey (1993) for a good practical guide to the analysis of qualitative data, and Strauss and Corbin (1990) for a more theoretical approach. The brief discussion below outlines a few general points that are particularly relevant to research into user perspectives.

Qualitative data analysis aims to go beyond describing participants' perspectives, to give a theoretical account of their strategies for managing situations. For example, Clarke, in Chapter 8, describes the way in which informal carers of people with dementia tried to cope by attempting to normalize their relationship with the dementing person. Formal carers, in contrast, saw themselves as managing inevitable decline.

The conclusions which are drawn from qualitative research will depend upon the researcher's interpretation of the data. Since the raw data is complex, e.g. transcripts of loosely structured dialogues between interviewer and users, interpretation must inevitably be subjective. The same data can be understood in several different ways. There is no one 'correct' way of interpreting qualitative data, but it is still necessary to ask questions about the reliability and validity of the researcher's conclusions (Kirk and Miller, 1986). How can we know that the researcher's account corresponds to at least some elements of users' views of the service, and so has validity at the level of meaning?

There can be no guarantees that interpretations of qualitative data are accurate. But there are useful steps that can be taken to test reliability and validity at the level of meaning, although each has limitations. Firstly, colleagues can be asked to examine the raw data, or a representative sample of it, blind to the principal researcher's interpretation, to see if they come to similar conclusions. However, many valid interpretations of the data are possible. Lack of correspondence does not necessarily imply that the first interpretation was 'wrong'. And both researchers may suffer from the same bias and produce similar (reliable) but invalid interpretations.

A second method of checking the validity of the data is to supply quotations from users in research reports that can be used by the reader to check the interpretation offered. Such checks are useful, but the reader can only consider the data supplied and has no way of knowing how it was selected. Even if the reader agrees with the researcher's interpretation, this may only show that both have the same bias.

The most important way of checking the researcher's interpretation of the data is to ask participants whether it is correct. Such feedback loops are an essential part of qualitative data collection. They may be implemented both informally during the main phase of data collection (Kirk and Miller, 1986) and after an initial report has been written. Informal feedback is possible with qualitative methods because data collection, analysis and redirection of questioning normally occur concurrently.

CONCLUSIONS

In this chapter, the value of researching user perspectives was considered from three angles, utilitarian, historical and methodological. It has been argued that their socialization, experience of health problems as work and lack of contact with other elements of overall health systems make it difficult for health professionals to see health care through the eyes of users.

Researching user perspectives is one way in which such perceptual 'gaps' may be lessened. However, the current wave of interest in researching user perspectives must be placed in a historical and political context. In Britain, such research appears, currently, to be part of an approach that aims to match services more closely to user needs while keeping power firmly in the hands of healthcare purchasers and providers.

Research into user perspectives is one way of consulting users without sharing power, but is subject to inescapable methodological problems associated with the definition of populations, the selection of samples, asking appropriate questions, obtaining valid answers and interpreting them correctly.

The chapters which follow explore user perspectives research in different sectors of community health care. The chapters illustrate a variety of methods, including participant observation (Chapter 3), diaries (Chapters 6 and 8), semi-structured qualitative interviewing (Chapters 3–10 and 12), surveys (Chapters 4, 8 and 13) and quasi-experiments (Chapters 5 and 11). The authors have attempted not to give idealized accounts but to describe the strengths and weaknesses of their research. It is hoped that the chapters that follow will give the reader an idea of what it means to research user perspectives.

CHAPTER 3

Accident and emergency departments in community health care

Geraldine S. Byrne

INTRODUCTION

Why include a chapter on accident and emergency departments?

A chapter which focuses on accident and emergency departments may seem an unusual inclusion in a book addressing users' perspectives on community health care. However, the accident and emergency department can be viewed as forming an integral part of community health care.

Accident and emergency is one of the few hospital departments to which patients can refer themselves without prior consultation with their GP or other health professional. In this respect, it is more akin to a primary health service than to most secondary sector provision. About 11.2 million new patients attended an accident and emergency department in England and Wales during 1991 (National Audit Office, 1992).

Freedom of access to accident and emergency departments has been enhanced by their traditional location within local communities (Cliff and Wood, 1986a; Walsh, 1990). However, increased centralization of departments in an effort to increase efficiency following the NHS and Community Care Act 1990 is reducing such local geographical links.

One consequence of open access is the varied range of problems that the department is exposed to. The typical workload includes people who present with alcohol- and drug-related problems; who have attempted suicide or suffered domestic violence; who complain of vague or chronic illnesses; and who simply seek reassurance and advice. Although most patients are discharged quickly, their health problems will often have longer-term social consequences, even if the medical condition is not serious, e.g. coping with a fracture. In such cases, an adequate response to both the antecedents and consequences of the patient's attendance at the accident and emergency department requires coordination with community services.

The scope of the chapter

Although the accident and emergency department is closely linked with the community, it remains, both bureaucratically and culturally, a hospital service. There is therefore a tension between the accident and emergency department as part of a hospital and as a community resource. This chapter will consider some of the implications of this dual role for patient care and will compare the perspectives of patients and staff in two departments. Methodological issues associated with the conduct of research into client and staff perspectives in the accident and emergency department will be discussed. Finally, the impact of current changes in health service provision on the nature and quality of accident and emergency department care will be considered.

BACKGROUND

Provider perspectives

Access to accident and emergency departments

Open access, however welcome to users, has been defined as a problem by providers of accident and emergency services since the inception of the NHS in 1948. The name change from casualty departments, following the Platt Report (1962), was intended to encourage patients to consult GPs where possible. Subsequently, several research reports documented the number and types of patients using the service 'inappropriately' (Dixon and Morris, 1971; Pease, 1973; O'Flanagan, 1976; Davison, Hildrey and Floyer, 1983; Cliff and Wood, 1986b). The incidence of 'inappropriate' attending appears to be increasing (Liggins, 1993; Sbaih, 1993) despite decades of provider concern.

'Inappropriate' attending, as described in this research, has included presenting with problems which could have been treated by a GP, misunderstanding the nature of the service provided and deliberate misuse. However, estimates of the extent of 'inappropriate attending' have ranged from 35% to 75% (Driscoll, Vincent and Wilkinson, 1987), suggesting definitional disagreements.

Most of these studies have been conducted by medical, nursing or administrative staff and have taken for granted the processes by which health professionals define attendance as 'inappropriate'. A more sociological approach (Roth, 1972; Jeffrey, 1979) has focused on staff attitudes towards 'deviant' patients. Gibson (1977) studied the ways in which patients are categorized and processed through the department. Hughes (1989) investigated the role of clerical staff as gatekeepers.

Functions of accident and emergency departments

There are in England some 235 main accident and emergency departments (National Audit Office, 1992). Their primary task is to care for ill or injured people quickly and at any time. Patients comprise:

- those with life-threatening illnesses and injuries, who require immediate medical assessment and may need resuscitation;
- those with serious illnesses or injuries, who require immediate medical assessment and may require admission to hospital;
- those with minor illnesses or injuries, who can often be quickly discharged after treatment.

The first group of patients make up only 1% of the total workload of the accident and emergency service (Warren, 1989). But the study described in this chapter suggests that these patients represent the main focus of staff interest. Clearly, the urgency and seriousness of these patients' conditions merit the priority with which they are treated. The Irving Report (1988) advocated the reorganization of accident and emergency services to more effectively meet their needs. Irving proposed that each Regional Health Authority should centralize accident and emergency department services so that human and technical resources could be pooled at one improved trauma centre.

Greater centralization may improve the technical quality of high technology, life-saving interventions (although it increases access time to the department). But it will also lead to the loss of a community resource and local alternatives need to be provided. The last part of Chapter 4 discusses the desire of one socially deprived group to have more, rather than less, locally based open access provision.

User perspectives

Despite the obvious importance of taking account of user perspectives in order to explain their attendance at accident and emergency departments, relatively little research has been carried out. The work which has been done suggests that patients' decisions to attend are influenced by their perceptions of the accident and emergency department and of their particular illness/injury. Instead of dismissing the attendance of a large proportion of patients as 'inappropriate', health providers need to understand their rationality.

Calnan (1984) compared the views of patients and staff about the seriousness of the patient's condition and found that patients were more likely than nurses to classify their injury as 'urgent'. This discrepancy could explain why health professionals judge so many patients to be attending inappropriately. It illustrates the separation of the worlds of health professionals and users discussed in Chapter 1.

It should not be assumed that patients are necessarily wrong when they differ from health professionals in their assessment of the seriousness of their condition or the appropriate location for treatment. Green and Dale (1992) found substantial differences between patients attending accident and emergency departments with primary care problems and those consulting GPs. The former were more likely to have injuries or symptoms of illness that they had not experienced previously and more likely to require further investigation. These findings suggest that a substantial proportion of patients have legitimate reasons for selecting the accident and emergency department rather than their GP.

Nguyen-Van-Tam and Baker (1992) compared admission rates among 103 patients who attended an accident and emergency department after consulting a GP with the same problem. The admission rate among patients who had not been referred to the accident and emergency department by their GP (34%) was slightly higher than the rate among patients who had been referred (28%). Patients' assessments of the seriousness of their problems were thus at least as good as those of their GPs.

The role of the nurse

Only a few studies have focused specifically on the activities of the nurse in the accident and emergency department (Wood, 1979; Clarke, 1982; Lewis and Bradbury, 1982; Toohey, 1984; Eaves, 1986) despite their potential role in meeting the social and psychological needs of patients. Wood (1979) found that nurse interactions with patients who had minor injuries were predominantly brief, task-centred and oriented to processing the patient through the department.

Many of the findings can be understood from the perspective of symbolic interactionism (Kelly and May, 1982). This approach emphasizes the influence of individuals' culturally mediated interpretations of the meaning of situations upon their behaviour. For example, Clarke (1982) compared patients' and nurses' views of patients' informational needs. Patients gave the highest priority to reassurance and explanation, while nurses felt that it was most important to teach preventative measures. The nurses' concern with prevention may be related to issues of open access, inappropriate attending and, ultimately, professional control. By stressing prevention they were suggesting, implicitly, that the patient ought to have avoided the injury in the first place. Patients, in contrast, were more concerned with the implications of the health problem.

Jeffrey (1979) concluded, as does the present study, that staff responded negatively to patients who were judged to be responsible for their own condition (e.g. drunks), or to be attending inappropriately. The present study found, however, that parents accompanying children were usually given prompt and friendly attention, even if the problem was trivial. Staff, then, appear to draw upon a quite complex stock of cultural knowledge when judging the legitimacy of patients' claims for their care.

METHODOLOGY

Introduction

The present study (Byrne, 1992) investigated sources of anxiety for patients aged over 18 in accident and emergency departments, their experiences in the department and the attitudes and communication pattern of nurses and other staff.

The research was carried out between 1987 and 1992 in two accident and emergency departments. Following an observational pilot study, it had three stages. Stage One employed structured interviews with 96 patients to identify sources of anxiety and to examine the relationships of anxiety to patient age, sex, seriousness of condition and department attended. In Stage Two, semi-structured interviews were conducted with 21 qualified nurses to explore their perceptions of their work. In Stage Three, the processing of 23 patients from admission to discharge was observed, with a focus on nurse–patient communication.

The sample

Choice of research sites and gatekeeping

The two accident and emergency departments in which the research was conducted were the only ones in the health authority in which the researcher was employed (as a staff nurse in another clinical setting in one of the hospitals). The role of colleague from another department who was undertaking research for an academic award provided a successful basis from which to establish good relations with nurses in the two departments.

Having negotiated access to the departments, the researcher had a 'captive audience' in the patients who attended the department and the nurses who worked there. Meetings were held with nurses in each department to explain the research, before observation took place or individuals were asked whether they were willing to participate. No nurse refused to take part in the research. The casualty officer was asked to inform the researcher if he thought any patient was too ill to take part, and consent was obtained from patients individually. No patients were excluded from or declined to take part in the main study. However, the consultant in one department refused permission for the researcher to observe interactions between doctors and patients, limiting the scope of Stage Three primarily to nurses and patients.

Selection of patients

So as to avoid selection bias in recruiting for the patient interview (Stage One) and observation (Stage Three), the next suitable patient was selected after the last patient being observed had been discharged or an interview had been completed.

Data was collected at different times during the day, so as to provide an element of time sampling. No night-time observations took place, as the conditions are so different, meriting a separate study.

Patient interviews (Stage One)

The patient interviews research design required a minimum of five patients in each of 16 subgroups based on combinations of age-group (under and over 40), sex, condition (minor versus serious or potentially serious) and department. A total of 96 patients were recruited.

Nurse interviews (Stage Two)

All qualified nurses working in the two departments not on permanent night duty (13 in one department and eight in the other) were interviewed.

Patient observation (Stage Three)

One week was spent observing patients in each department (10 in one department and 13 in the other). Only two patients fitted into the 'young major' category (people aged under 40 with serious or potentially serious conditions), a relatively unusual group, and it was not possible to extend the observation period in order to obtain more cases. Both were female, one from each department. Conclusions about this group must be regarded as particularly tentative, although findings about 'what exists' (Walker, 1982, p. 3) do not depend upon sample size.

Methods

Introduction

The research utilized qualitative and quantitative methods of data collection and analysis eclectically, depending upon their appropriateness for particular purposes. Quantitative data on patient anxieties obtained in the Stage One structured patient interviews was used to obtain a general, representative picture of the nature and extent of patient anxieties. Intensive qualitative interviews with nurses in Stage Two were used to explore the ways in which they interpreted their roles and their views of patients. The observational data obtained in Stage Three was analysed both quantitatively and qualitatively. Quantitative behaviour counts were used to assess who communicated what to whom. Qualitative analysis provided an insight into the ways in which patients were processed through the department.

Data collection at each research stage was guided by analysis of the results of previous stages. When interviewing nurses in Stage Two, the researcher had already identified major patient concerns such as the social consequences of the accident or injury. She had concluded that nurses were most interested in dramatic cases of major trauma or life-threatening illness rather than the social consequences of mundane medical problems. This difference in orientation provided a context for the observation of nurse–patient interaction in Stage Three. For example, strategies that nurses employed to close off patient-initiated discussions of their own concerns could be identified.

Stage One: patient interviews

For Stage One, a structured interview schedule was used with 96 patients, in order to obtain an initial quantitative representation of patient anxieties. It was also possible to relate measured anxiety levels to patient age, sex, seriousness of condition and department attended.

The schedule asked patients to rate the amount of anxiety that they felt about a series of items associated with the accident or emergency and their stay in the department. It was based on the schedule used by Danis (1984), modified slightly for a British context. In the light of pilot work, questions were added covering anxiety about relatives not knowing where the patient was or what was happening.

Patient interviews indicated that the main sources of anxiety for patients were associated with the social implications of their illness/injury and not knowing or being unable to control what would happen to them in the department.

Stage Two: nurse interviews

Observation undertaken during the pilot study suggested that patient anxieties were not usually addressed by staff. In Stage Two, nurses' perceptions of their work and of patients were investigated, using semi-structured interviews. Interviews were organized around a list of topics, but these were not covered in any prearranged order, and points which respondents raised were fully explored.

Interviews, which lasted 40–60 minutes, were conducted confidentially in sister's office, taped, transcribed and analysed for recurring themes.

The researcher found during the pilot study that it was very difficult to talk to nurses about events observed at the time they occurred, or immediately afterwards, as the nurse was either engaged in the task in hand or had moved on to another. Having a period set aside for the interview enabled nurses to reflect upon their work without interruption or distraction. On the other hand, their recall of events might be affected by faulty memory or the desire to present a favourable picture.

Stage Three: observation of nurse–patient interaction

Stage Three involved observation of nurse–patient interactions, in order to assess the extent to which patient anxieties were addressed. Selected patients were followed through the ward from admission to discharge. The researcher attempted to minimize reactivity by communicating with the patient as little as possible and by adopting an unobtrusive position, e.g. in the corner of a cubicle. She soon became 'part of the furniture'.

The unit of analysis was the topic, defined as a particular subject discussed between a member of staff and the patient or relative. Each topic was coded in terms of the time the interaction took, who initiated it and the topic type. Topic types were coded from a list of 17, established from two pilot observations. They included, for example, waiting times, what would happen to the patient, specific procedures and impact on daily life. Space was left for qualitative comments.

Issues in data collection

The main issues in data collection concerned the impact of the researcher upon the activities of the department. The need to avoid interfering with the delivery of care sometimes affected data collection. For example, to avoid interrupting busy nurses, interviews with them had to be conducted at a time and place they found convenient.

A second issue was the risk of reactivity. Nurses may have behaved differently in the presence of the researcher, for example by appearing more busy than usual. However, their increasing familiarity with the researcher and need to concentrate on the job in hand probably minimized this problem.

During the pilot study it was found that patients who would otherwise have been alone while awaiting investigations, treatment or results appreciated the presence and interest of the researcher. A more distant approach was therefore adopted for later observation. But to have been rigidly uncommunicative would have seemed false and would probably have proved counter-productive. A balance had to be struck. The researcher responded politely to conversations initiated by patients and their relatives. As a by-product, this strategy provided useful contextual material about what patients were thinking while they were being observed.

A more general issue was the problem of being a nurse researching other nurses. Not working in an accident and emergency department helped the researcher to be objective. But it felt, at times, uncomfortable to be critical of colleagues who were doing a demanding job. What the study does suggest, however, is that our priorities, as nurses, do not always correspond with those of our patients.

RESULTS

Processing patients

The patient's encounter with the hospital had an organized structure with a beginning (admission), middle (diagnostic procedures and treatment) and end (discharge into the community or another hospital ward).

Admission: defining the patient role

Part of the control nurses exercised over patients was achieved by the confirmation of the individual as patient. Admission to the accident and emergency department involved a number of procedures, particularly for those with more serious conditions, that had the instrumental purpose of preparing the patient to be seen by the doctor but may also have had the expressive function of confirming the person in the role of patient (Goffman, 1961).

On arrival in the department, such patients would be helped to change from outdoor clothes into a gown. The patient's belongings would be packed up and placed on the trolley on which he or she would be asked to lie. Temperature, pulse and blood pressure would then be taken and a brief history of the condition recorded.

Nurses perceived problems, expressed in the Stage Two interviews, in achieving control, particularly over patients who had minor complaints. They felt unable to exercise as much control over their patients as was possible on other hospital wards.

> It's not like on the wards where you strip them down, and put them in their pyjamas, and immediately become in charge, whereas here they more or less meet you on an equal footing. (Nurse)

Another nurse saw accident and emergency patients as straddling two 'worlds', the hospital and the community, worlds which, by implication, she saw as widely separated.

When you think how other nurses look after their patients really, like, for example, I know everyone has to be undressed, to be admitted to hospital, stuck in a bed, and you've got to do this at certain times, and all this, that and the other. Well our patients just wouldn't wear that, you know. It wouldn't wash with them because, of course **they've got one foot in the outside world. They're not actually admitted.** (Nurse – author's emphasis)

Managing the stay

Following admission, nurses reinforced the message that the patient should be passive and undemanding by appearing permanently busy. Nurses described a strategy of 'popping', 'dashing' or 'nipping' in on patients to deliver care. Nurses acknowledged that this strategy was, at times, consciously employed.

Well they soon get the message that we're busy. (Nurse)

One reason nurses gave for this behaviour was that they wished to remain in a state of readiness in case an emergency was admitted. By avoiding remaining in rooms with patients, the nurses fulfilled their aims of maintaining a general surveillance and being able to respond to needs as they arose. They also saw this strategy as a means of managing the frequently conflicting demands upon their time.

This approach may enable nurses to maintain their availability to deal with immediate physical problems, but is unlikely to be successful as a means of identifying and dealing with patients' concerns. Indeed, the strategy was an effective way in which to convey to patients that the nurses were not to be troubled with unnecessary questions.

Communication breakdowns were at times the result. For example, one young woman, admitted with abdominal pain, was very anxious about what might be wrong with her. After she had had an X-ray, the casualty officer decided that she needed a scan. The patient only discovered that she was to have a scan when the auxiliary nurse said that the porter would be coming shortly to fetch her. While waiting in X-ray the patient expressed her concern to the researcher.

If there was anything wrong with the X-ray they would have told me, wouldn't they? (Patient)

After the scan had been performed she was still not told why it had been considered necessary. Because communication with staff was disjointed, the patient's worries were not identified or dealt with. She had, in fact, only been given a scan as a final check because the X-ray had been found to be normal.

Several patients were observed to express concern to relatives or companions about the social implications of their illness/injury, for example what would happen if they were admitted, or how they would cope if discharged. Such fears were rarely communicated to nurses. The brief duration of encounters with nurses, associated with their strategy of 'popping in' and their focus on physical care, seemed to discourage patients from raising such concerns.

For example, one self-employed businessman who had broken his leg, and had been told to 'stay off it', was very concerned about the effect this would have on his work. He commented to his wife:

Stay off it? That's very easy to say. (Patient)

However, his concern was not disclosed to the nurses.

Patient anxiety about having to stay in hospital tended to be ignored, in favour of a medical necessity which was presumed to take priority.

I hope they won't be keeping me in. (Elderly patient)

We don't know at the moment. Obviously we won't keep you in unless we have to. It's in everyone's interest to get you home if we can. But obviously we can't do that unless you're well enough. (Nurse)

This patient was later observed to repeat her concern to the nurse, but the reason for her anxiety was not explored.

Social factors generally were given limited attention, even when they were directly related to the cause of admission. A female patient, for example, revealed on admission that she had been beaten by her partner and that, during the incident, his dog had bitten her. During her time in the department the care of the woman centred on the treatment of the bite. The circumstances surrounding its occurrence were not discussed.

One reason for the nurses' lack of attention to the social causes and consequences of patients' injuries may have been their sense of powerlessness in the face of social problems. As one of the nurses caring for the female victim of domestic violence stated:

It's a shame what happened, but unless they're prepared to do something for themselves, there's nothing we can do to help them. (Nurse)

However, it is possible that some concerns could have been dealt with, perhaps through an improved system of referral to other agencies.

Discharge

Of the patients observed in Stage Three, 19 were discharged home and four admitted to hospital. Communication with 'minor' patients at this stage was predominantly about medical procedures. One nurse identified a gap between nurse and patient perspectives.

A small cut on the finger could be nothing to us, but could be horrendous to them ... and we tend to overlook that. (Nurse)

'Minor' patients seemed satisfied with the discharge information they received and only two asked questions about going back to work. Two further patients expressed worries about going back to work to the researcher, but did not mention their concern to any nurse. There seems to have been an implicit understanding on both sides that there was nothing that nurses could do to help and that managing the social consequences of the accident or emergency was not their problem.

Patients with more serious conditions were either admitted to hospital (four patients) or discharged home (five patients). The patients who were admitted, including the elderly person who had expressed concern to nurses, were given little opportunity to discuss their feelings or any practical problems.

Mrs X, you're going to ward 7. (Nurse)

Am I? I was hoping to be able to go home. (Patient)

The doctor said she's not happy for you to go home. You're not really managing are you? And you won't be able to manage at all now. (Nurse)

The patient made no response to this demonstration of professional power, which was not based on any discussion with her about home circumstances.

Nurses' and patients' perceptions of the department

Comparison of data from the nurse and patient interviews and the observational material revealed a contrast between nurses' and patients' perspectives on the patient's presence in the accident and emergency department. The concern which, in the Stage One interviews, patients most frequently mentioned as causing them anxiety was not being able to carry on their usual activities. Anxiety about this item was expressed by 81% (68) of the 96 patients who were interviewed. More than half the sample acknowledged anxiety about being unable to control, or not knowing, what would happen to them in the department, having to undergo an uncomfortable procedure and feeling pain. Patients were thus at least as concerned about the psychological and social consequences of admission as with their physical condition and its treatment.

Nurses, however, were preoccupied with immediate physical care and the organization of the patient's stay in the department. Of 156 topics addressed by nurses to patients in the Stage Three observational study, 60% were concerned with details of care including admission and discharge, what would happen in the department, directions where to go, waiting times and care of dressings. The nature of the medical condition was the focus of a further 19% of nurse initiated topics. Only 4% of nurse-initiated topics were concerned with the patient's psychological and social needs, including anxieties, impact on daily life and pain.

During Stage Three, patients only initiated 19 topics with nurses in total (compared with the 156 initiated by nurses) and 13 of the 23 Stage Three patients initiated no topics with nurses. Of the 19 topics which patients initiated with nurses, six were about anxieties, impact on daily life and pain. Thus, about a third of an admittedly small sample of patient-initiated communications was about the psychological and social effects of the accident or emergency, compared with only 4% of those initiated by nurses (see above). The topics initiated thus reflect the differing priorities of nurses and patients.

The type of communication occurring between nurses and patients reflected the nurses' view of their role. The Stage Two nurse interviews suggested that many nurses had been attracted to working in the accident and emergency department to get away from what they saw as routine and uneventful ward work.

> When I first qualified, I staffed on a male surgical ward for five months. I found it fulfilling, but also very boring, because you have set routines, set operating days and so forth, whereas casualty is totally different. You don't know what's coming through the doors next. Although you have a set routine to a certain extent, it's just totally unpredictable. (Nurse)

Another feature of their work which nurses valued was the opportunity to care for 'major trauma' patients.

> Most people who work in casualty like the excitement of, you know, you get a lot of minor stuff, but it's the major stuff that keeps people's interest, you know. (Nurse)

However, much of their work was not of this nature, but involved caring for patients with minor and non-urgent illnesses and injuries.

> It's more sprained ankles than anything else. (Nurse)

While nurses accepted patients with minor injuries, they did get exasperated with the number of 'inappropriate' attenders they had to deal with.

> You just don't realize the amount of tripe that comes through the door. (Nurse)

Drunks and regulars were the most strongly disliked patients. But those who attended the department 'inappropriately' for other reasons, typically with what the nurses perceived as an unacceptably minor or old injury, were also disapproved of.

They forget they've got GPs, or they don't like their GP, so they think they've got the right to walk in here and be seen. Well it doesn't work like that, and if you try and explain to them they get annoyed, because they've trailed up here. (Nurse)

However, patients with recent injuries, however slight, did have a right to be seen, a fact which the nurses sometimes regretted.

If people come in with a new injury today, we've got to see them, unfortunately. (Nurse)

This nurse perspective conflicted with the views of patients, a high proportion of whom expressed anxieties about their condition and its consequences in the Stage One interviews.

Nurses, because of their orientation towards emergencies, did not regard it as their responsibility to address the wider social and behavioural context of health problems. In the case of the drunks, the nurses' solution was, as far as possible, to ignore them.

The drunks I don't like looking after at all – I think there should be a place for them. It's not right that they should come in here, and they're shouting abuse, and just carrying on. They all have to be seen because they may have done something, so they have to be seen, but we try and ignore them, to tell you the honest truth. (Nurse)

However, the drunks and other 'regulars' were likely to reappear because their problems were not addressed, for example, by offering them referral to other agencies.

DISCUSSION

Because nurses defined the role of the accident and emergency department primarily in terms of dealing with major trauma, thus adopting an implicit medical model, they largely failed to address the psychological and social needs of patients who were seen as blameworthy (e.g. drunks), or as having run of the mill, uninteresting medical problems. The social and behavioural factors leading to regular attendance were not usually discussed. Patients were not offered referral to other agencies who might have been able to provide longer-term help. This is regrettable, because patients may be most open to advice about chronic problems such as alcohol misuse or domestic violence at points of time at which their 'careers' are punctuated by accidents or emergencies.

Patients whose illnesses or injuries would obviously have a major impact on their life were either admitted to the hospital or discharged home with district nurse and social services support. Other patients, with minor injuries, could easily continue their normal activities with, at most, minor disruption. However, a third group of patients had conditions which were not medically serious but which made them dependent upon support from others (e.g. a fracture). It was assumed that these patients could cope with support from family and friends. The social dimensions of their condition were not usually considered. Accident and emergency department staff were oriented towards the medical causes of impairment rather than towards disability or handicap.

There is a need for community services to be developed to fill this gap and for links between accident and emergency departments and existing services to be improved. Part of the problem may be due to a lack of knowledge on the part of accident and emergency department staff about resources available in the community. In one area, aftercare has been found to be inadequate even for the elderly, a particularly vulnerable group (West Birmingham Community Health Council, 1990). Recommendations included the routine collection of information about home circumstances, social support and improvements in community health and social services. Townsend *et al.* (1992) found that providing elderly patients discharged from hospital with additional community support led to a significant reduction in emergency readmissions.

The accident and emergency department should be seen as part of the community which it serves. Health problems need to be understood from patients' perspectives. Improved links between accident and emergency departments and other services are needed if the human antecedents and consequences of accidents and emergencies are to be addressed. One way to improve liaison is to locate primary health care services within accident and emergency departments (Green, Dale and Glucksman, 1991).

Another policy which may improve the response of accident and emergency departments to patients' social and psychological needs is the introduction of nurse practitioners (Morris, Head and Volkar, 1989; Woolich, 1992). It is perhaps even more important that other current changes do not undermine the present availability of services. The trend towards centralization of trauma units may threaten provision to local communities. In order to prevent a reduction in the accessibility and quality of care available, it is essential that centralized services are replaced by suitable alternative provision, such as minor injury units and nurse-run clinics, which can effectively meet the needs of the local community (see the last part of Chapter 4).

Patients' views of GPs

Bob Heyman

INTRODUCTION

This chapter aims to compare two research projects, quantitative and qualitative, into patients' perceptions of GPs. It is not suggested that one is 'better' than the other, or even that there is a clear dividing line between qualitative and quantitative work, which can usefully complement each other (Silverman, 1985; Bryman, 1988).

Both projects were funded by Family Health Service Authorities (FHSAs) and the author was involved in design and analysis. The Patient Survey (PS) was sponsored jointly by an FHSA, Community Health Council and Local Medical Committee responsible for a mixed rural/urban county with substantial areas of industrial decay and high unemployment. Questionnaires were posted to a random sample of named individuals in 1991/2. Subsequently, volunteer practices were surveyed individually.

The Health Needs Project (HNP) was carried out in 1992/3 and used focus groups to investigate qualitatively the perceived health needs of residents of one of the poorest parts of Tyne and Wear.

The two projects are not fully comparable because of differences in their target populations and research focus. Nevertheless, comparisons are instructive, and will be drawn out in the Discussion section.

BACKGROUND

Surveys initiated by community health councils have become popular in recent years as a method of evaluating consumer responses to GP services (Tameside and Glossop CHC, 1987; Williamson, 1988; Yarde and Forest, 1989; West Cumbria CHC, 1990). Surveys also allow patient satisfaction to be related to other variables, but relationships which have been found with age and social class tend to be weak and inconsistent (Fox and Storms, 1981).

Surveys have shown a high overall level of consumer satisfaction, although less so for information giving than for other aspects of care such as examining and prescribing (e.g. West Cumbria CHC, 1990). Research initiated by academics has yielded similar positive findings (e.g. Patrick, Scrivens and Charlton, 1983), although patients again consistently identify communication problems (Simpson *et al.*, 1991). However, in the absence of more detailed qualitative data, the meaning of these findings is problematic.

The use of satisfaction surveys has been widely criticized (Fitzpatrick and Hopkins, 1983). Two related criticisms are particularly relevant to this chapter and to the book. Firstly, survey questions tend to reflect medical agendas rather than patient concerns. Secondly, such questions require patients to generalize in ways which may not be meaningful for them and which may be only weakly related to their concrete experience (Calnan, 1988).

Loosely structured focus groups are not an effective tool for assessing individual perspectives or making specific comparisons. But they are sensitive to the common concerns of group members, concerns which are likely to surface as conversation topics. By stimulating ideas and anecdotes (Hedges, 1985) and encouraging dialogue between participants (Kitzinger, 1994) they generate the concrete details of patient perspectives.

Questionnaires initiated by providers of medical services tend to reflect their priorities. For example, there were 20 questions in the PS about the adequacy of the waiting and consulting rooms but this issue was never mentioned by focus group members in the HNP. Doctors' perceived ability to diagnose was not assessed in the PS because the research commissioners believed that patients were not capable of assessing diagnostic ability. Some group members in the HNP apparently did not share this belief and made scathing comments about their doctor's poor (perceived) diagnostic skills. Their main concern was the development of services outside GP practices, e.g. locally based counselling and first aid. Questions about unmet need and alternatives services were not asked in the PS.

THE PATIENT SURVEY

Methodology

The sample

The sampling frame was the FHSA Patient Register. Unregistered patients were thus excluded. Questionnaires were posted to an unstratified random sample of 1010 named individuals.

Where the named person was unable to complete the questionnaire, because he or she was too young or infirm, another member of the household was asked to fill it in to reflect the named person's views as far as possible. Over half (54%) of the 172 other-completed questionnaires were filled in on behalf of someone aged under 10. One respondent declined to comment because she was a baby! The accuracy of these questionnaires (22% of the 800 completed) is problematic. However, analysis with and without other-completed questionnaires did not appreciably affect the conclusions of the research.

Two follow-up questionnaires were sent to non-respondents. The final response rate, 79%, was high for a postal survey, although the first questionnaire was returned by only 46% (463) of those approached. The high eventual response rate perhaps reflects the public-spirited, altruistic feelings which people in Britain have traditionally felt for the NHS. Higher response rates have been found for postal surveys sent out by Family Practitioner Committees than for those sent out by a research organization (Jacoby, 1990). The questionnaire appealed for participation with the words: 'Please read these notes. Now help us to help you!'

The 21% of the sample who were not represented may have had significantly different attitudes. For example, the least satisfied might have been less willing to participate. One advantage of a formal survey involving a probability sample is that it is possible to check the representativeness of the sample in at least some respects, as illustrated below. This was done firstly by comparing sample estimates of the age/sex distribution with data provided for the population by the FHSA and secondly by comparing those who completed the first, second and third questionnaire. The assumption behind this comparison is that 'late returners' will be more like non-respondents than those who return the first requested questionnaire (Drane, 1991).

Younger respondents, excluding the 0–10 age group who did not complete the questionnaires for themselves, were significantly under-represented in comparison with the FHSA database and were more likely to be 'late' responders, suggesting that they were less likely to participate than older groups. Late responding was also significantly associated with the conventionally defined 'head of household' having a lower occupational socioeconomic status, as assessed by the Registrar General's classification.

It will be shown below that younger age and lower socioeconomic status were associated with greater dissatisfaction with GP services. Since these groups were less likely to participate, the results probably overestimate patient satisfaction.

Methods

The questionnaire covered getting to the surgery, services offered and used, doctors' accessibility and professional conduct, the helpfulness of receptionists, the waiting and consulting rooms and demographic information. There were a few questions about nurses, health visitors and midwives. Most questions were 'closed', asking respondents to choose from a small number of possible replies, but comments were requested at various points.

Use of standard FHSA patient code numbers allowed the questionnaire data to be linked to information in the FHSA database about each patient's practice, including size, the number of doctors, their age and sex and trainer and fundholding status. In order to protect patient confidentiality, patient names were known only to the FHSA, while the database which linked FHSA and questionnaire data could be accessed only by University of Northumbria staff.

Results

Descriptive data on patient perceptions of GP practices

For reasons of space, only a small number of findings will be briefly mentioned. Percentages given below are based on the total numbers (shown in parentheses) who responded and were not 'uncertain'. The maximum possible sample size was 800.

Over 90% of respondents felt that the doctor was normally good at listening, explaining and examining, and were happy with the way in which the doctor prescribed medicines (with over 700 making a judgement in each case). The percentage who felt that the doctor was normally good at explaining things is rather higher than the proportion rating the doctor good at giving information in other studies (see above), perhaps because of differences in question wording.

About 90% felt that surgery hours were convenient ($n = 747$), and that consultation length was adequate ($n = 747$). But other aspects of access received more frequent criticism. The length of routine delays for a midweek appointment with any doctor were considered unreasonable by 25% of the sample ($n = 683$). Only 54% ($n = 794$) found it very easy to get to the surgery, and only 60% ($n = 775$) rated their general impression of the waiting room as good.

In terms of relationships with staff, only 66% ($n = 738$) rated the relationship with their doctor as good. Receptionist helpfulness was rated good by 50% of the sample ($n = 742$). These findings suggest further questions about patient expectations which cannot be answered from the survey data. What expectations did patients have of doctors and why did they see receptionists as unhelpful?

Patient perspectives and other variables

Differences in patient perspectives were related to a variety of demographic variables and variables describing features of the practice (practice variables).

The demographic variables considered in this chapter are patient age, sex, urban/rural residence and 'head of household' socioeconomic status, based on the Registrar General's classification. To simplify the analysis, respondents were classified as having either non-manual (professional and skilled non-manual) or manual occupations. This classification was a crude one, intended to give no more than a rough indicator of socioeconomic circumstances.

The practice variables included the size of the practice (number of patients registered), the patient–doctor ratio, the average age of the doctors and fundholding and trainer status. The research took place just as fundholding was being implemented. The one difference found (better waiting rooms in fundholding practices) probably reflects a difference in the kinds of practice that became early fundholders, e.g. that they were larger, rather than being a result of fundholding.

The analysis presented in Table 4.1 used the technique of logistic regression, available in SPSS/PC, to relate binary variables (e.g. was the doctor rated good at listening or not?) to practice and demographic variables. Logistic regression has the advantage over traditional techniques such as crosstabulation and chi-square of allowing the effects of several independent variables to be considered simultaneously. Logistic regression will select the variables which, in combination, are most closely associated with the dependent variable.

Techniques of multivariate analysis, including logistic regression, have a number of limitations. They are essentially exploratory. With a large number of independent variables, some combinations are likely to have statistically significant relationships with the dependent variable just by chance. When independent variables are themselves related, small chance differences can determine which ones are selected. Statistically significant relationships are not necessarily causal and even the direction of causality can be problematic.

Examples of the kinds of relationship found are presented in Table 4.1.

The 'r' column in Table 4.1 provides a coefficient which measures the strength of the relationship between the patient perception and independent variable. A coefficient of 1 would indicate that one variable could be predicted completely by the other. The strongest relationships, shown in the table, have coefficients of about 0.2 (associated with patient age), indicating weak relationships, even though they are highly significant statistically, due to the large size of the sample. Patients could only be included in an analysis if information was available on all variables included in the analysis. The 'ns' in Table 4.1 show that substantial numbers were excluded, threatening the representativeness of the relationships discovered.

Although the relationships shown in Table 4.1 were weak, there were clear patterns in the data. Patient sex was associated with none of the variables. Less favourable evaluations were more likely from younger patients, those with manual social class backgrounds and those from urban areas (although rural residents were less likely to find it very easy to get to the surgery). Surprisingly, further analysis showed that the relationship between manual social class and finding it harder to get to the surgery was statistically independent of access to a car. One possible explanation, discussed below in relation to the HNP, is that surgeries are less likely to be located in poorer areas.

Table 4.1 Statistically significant predictors of patient perceptions of GP practices – examples of analyses using logistic regression

Patient perception	Variables significantly associated at < 0.05 level	r	n
Doctor normally good at listening	Rural residence	0.14	542
	Younger doctors	0.11	
	Lower patient–doctor ratio	0.13	
Doctor normally good at explaining	Trainer practice	0.15	537
Doctor normally good at examining	Trainer practice	0.10	522
Surgery hours convenient	Older patients	0.16	551
	Higher patient–doctor ratio	0.13	
Days wait for routine appointment reasonable	Fewer patients	0.15	503
	Non-manual social class	0.09	
Very easy to get to surgery	Fewer patients	0.10	556
	Younger doctors	0.08	
	Urban residence	0.07	
	Non-manual social class	0.06	
Relationship with doctor good	Older patients	0.20	548
	Non-manual social class	0.08	
Receptionist helpfulness good	Older patients	0.21	549
	Fewer patients	0.08	
	Non-manual social class	0.08	

Patients were less likely to be satisfied in one or more areas (of which only examples are shown in Table 4.1) with non-trainer and non-fundholding practices, those with older doctors and those with more patients. Practice size (more patients) was associated with perceived delays to see the doctor, difficulty in getting to the surgery and receptionist unhelpfulness. However, patient–doctor ratios were not a factor in any of these relationships, suggesting that the problems in large practices might be organizational.

Patients attending practices with higher patient–doctor ratios were more likely to criticize doctors' listening skills, but were more likely to be satisfied with the convenience of surgery hours. Perhaps these doctors had to keep longer hours in order to see all their patients!

Practice surveys

The FHSA offered doctors the opportunity to have the survey repeated in their own practice. Six out of 48 practices in the country chose to have their practice surveyed, with questionnaires sent to at least 600 patients in each. The results have been fed back, confidentially, to GPs in the form of tables comparing patient perspectives on the practice, question by question, with the average for the entire county. The surveys provide a detailed profile of the strengths and weaknesses of the practice as seen by patients, and allow standardized comparisons to be made. For example, in one practice, otherwise evaluated very favourably, patients rated toys for children less favourably than in other practices and young women were less aware of family planning services.

The profiles of the six practices which have chosen to have surveys suggest that gatekeeping processes were at work in their self-selection. Older patients and those from non-manual occupations were over-represented in the practice populations, compared with the average for the county. In general, the practices, particularly the doctors, were evaluated significantly more favourably than average, even when the tendency of older people and those from non-manual backgrounds to give more favourable ratings were controlled for statistically. Retrospective analysis showed that doctors in practices which subsequently opted to have an individual survey were evaluated more favourably in the original survey, although the differences were not statistically significant, perhaps due to smaller numbers. Thus, it would appear that the practices which chose to be surveyed were the ones that patients would be least likely to criticize.

THE HEALTH NEEDS PROJECT

Introduction

The research was initiated by a women's community group who had a clear agenda, to provide ammunition to support their case for a health and community centre for the deprived estate in which they lived. The researchers had some anxiety at the start of the project that they would end up merely repeating the views of the converted as part of a worthy propaganda exercise. As will be explained below, great efforts were taken to try to obtain representative views from the whole community.

The estate which was the focus for the research is situated about five miles from the centre of an urban area within Tyne and Wear and has about 9000 residents. The bus journey to the nearest city centre, with its shopping and leisure facilities, takes about 30 minutes each way and costs over £1.50 per adult for the return trip, beyond the means of families surviving on state benefit. The estate is one of the most socially deprived in North-East England. According to the 1991 census, 64% of households did not have use of a car, the unemployment rate among economically active persons was 24% for men and 14% for women and the long-term sickness rate among persons aged under 60 was 13%.

The standard of housing is generally reasonable, and there is an ongoing programme of improvement. But residents are trapped on the estate by lack of affordable transport, while amenities within walking distance are virtually non-existent. There are small shops but no supermarket and little in the way of parks, leisure and recreation facilities other than pubs and clubs. The only health facility on the estate is a small pharmacy. There are no health or welfare centres, doctors, dentists, opticians or chiropodists within easy walking distance.

Methodology

The sample

The community group initially sent out questionnaires about health needs, after a public meeting, but received a response rate of only 2%.

It was then decided to try to recruit focus groups and to offer residents £10 for participation, plus child care and transport, if needed. The response rate, based on letters returned by a random sample of 400 households, was 3%! The 12 people who were recruited were used to run two pilot groups, one of adults aged 25 and over and one of (mildly) disabled people.

The women in the community group, at their own suggestion, began house-to-house recruiting within a random sample of households. A letter was sent first, inviting residents to reply, post-free, if they did not want someone to call and invite them to participate. Of a random sample of 100 households, 10 returned a slip refusing to be visited and 12 letters were returned unopened for other reasons. The volunteers were able to visit 65 of the remaining households and to make a contact in 40. From these 40 households, 30 individuals were recruited. They recommended other people on the estate. Together with local contacts, a final sample of 127 was obtained of whom 113, 35 males and 78 females, showed up for the group discussions. Without the 'insider' help of the community group, recruitment of such a sample might have proved impossible.

A total of 16 groups were formed from the sample, two of each of the following eight kinds of group: adults; parents with young children; carers; over 60s; the unemployed; the disabled; and four single-sex groups of boys and girls aged 12–15 and 16–19.

The sample was not representative of residents. Women were over-represented in the groups whose sex was not predetermined. There were no males in the carer groups, or the groups of parents with children. The researchers had hoped to involve moderately or severely disabled people, but those recruited were only mildly disabled. They seemed little different to other adults, given the poor level of health of residents on the estate.

Methods

A short interview schedule was tested on two pilot groups. The schedule contained open questions covering the meaning of 'health', personal health, use of health services, the health of the estate and views of the government's health priorities. These questions were used as a stimulus to encourage group discussion.

Given the qualitative nature of the methodology, interviewers had discretion to ask follow-up questions which depended on the content of the discussion, but were asked to avoid leading questions as far as possible. The main interviewer, employed for the research, conducted 11 of the remaining focus group sessions, with the rest led by others involved in the research, for scheduling reasons. The focus groups took place between November 1992 and April 1993.

Each group lasted about 90 minutes and was tape-recorded using a special multidirectional microphone; 13 of these interviews were professionally transcribed, generating 400 pages of discussion. Three interviews could not be transcribed due to an intermittent technical fault which was eventually traced to (new) tapes that had been overwound. Interview notes suggest that the inclusion of these three groups (one carer, one disabled and one parents of young children) would not have affected the conclusions.

The data were analysed by developing a list of themes and recording the themes associated with each topic in the conversation into a database, together with short notes and a reference to the group and the page(s) in the transcript. A separate listing was then printed for each theme, providing a brief overview of respondents' views. These were used to develop an analysis of residents' perceived health needs, examples of which are given in the next section.

A detailed report was produced for the FHSA, and discussed with them at one of their regular meetings. A summary of this report was given to all who had participated in the research. Residents were invited to an open meeting to discuss the results.

Results

Introduction

The views of the different groups complemented each other strongly, reflecting a common experience of multiple deprivation on the estate. Therefore, the comparative method (Strauss and Corbin, 1990, p. 62) was not appropriate. The findings are presented as a composite picture of residents' views of health and health care.

Residents' views will be discussed in relation to three related issues: firstly, their concepts of health; secondly, their perceptions of barriers to health; and thirdly, their view about the future development of health care.

Concepts of health

When asked what health meant to them, most group members replied in concrete terms, e.g. mentioning smoking or diet. Abstract definitions were less common. They included positive concepts of health, health as a resource, being active and coping.

Only two group members, both elderly, expressed positive concepts of health.

Try to look on a happy side of life, and I think you can help it [control your own health]. (Elderly woman)

Health as well-being was more often viewed from the opposite direction, poor mental health explained by poverty and social pressure.

Money. Stress. Families. Pressures. Stress. I mean it's very rare you see anybody up here running around happy as sunbeams, is it? (Woman carer)

A few group members saw health as a resource enabling them to achieve life goals, the WHO (1986) definition.

If you've got good health you've got practically nine-tenths of everything haven't you? Because, without your health, you can't do anything. (Adult woman)

Some respondents related health to being active, but in a negative sense, as social conditions were seen as leading to inactivity for people on the estate. Inactivity was associated with unemployment, lack of accessible leisure facilities, cost and fear, particularly for women and elderly people, of walking on the estate. Inactivity was seen as having various effects on health, including boredom, family stress, poor fitness, smoking, alcohol consumption and drug-taking. The quotation below illustrates some of these themes.

I never let my son out. I mean on the dark nights.... And there's nowhere else to take him, because I wouldn't walk about in the dark. (Unemployed woman)

So there you are. Detrimental to two healths. The mother who's got them kids around the house, and the bairns cannot get out in the fresh air. (Unemployed man)

Most group members defined health in terms of specific issues such as a healthy diet, not smoking or consuming excessive alcohol, exercise and, among young people, avoiding drugs. Mothers of older children and girls aged 12–19 were also concerned about avoiding unplanned pregnancies and about safe sex.

> Take care of your body. Eat the right stuff. Take some form of exercise. You should have a regular visit to your health centre so you can have the check-ups. (Unemployed man)

Such definitions imply an acceptance of the official line on health promotion. This line was only rarely rejected, as below, at least in the context of group discussions about health.

> Some people can smoke all their lives, and live to a ripe old age. (Woman carer)

Most group members were concerned that they smoked, ate too many chips or did not exercise. However, they explained these behaviours in terms of adverse social circumstances rather than individual choice. Thus their apparently simple behavioural definitions of health were part of a more elaborated social model of health.

> But when I left there [employment] ... I had nowt to do during the day. And so you were sitting there, and you had a cup of tea, and you can't be bothered – 'Oh, I think I'll have a fag'.... And then you're addicting yourself to it. (Unemployed woman)

> But, health-food-wise, it would cost you a fortune to buy the stuff that you were supposed to eat.... So, basically, they just get an apple and an orange, and the rest of it is mostly fried stuff. (Young adult woman)

> Or you could take drugs, like if your mum and dad, say, split up. Like, the kids could turn to sniffing or something daft like that. (Girl aged 12–15)

Barriers to health

Group members' problems, as they saw them, can be visualized as three concentric circles. The core circle, at the root of their problems, was the double demon of poverty and unemployment. The second circle represents lack of community resources, e.g. supermarkets, parks, leisure facilities. This lack prevented people from compensating for the effects of poverty and unemployment, or made things worse. The outer circle represents inaccessible and inappropriate primary health care services which failed to put right health problems arising from poverty, unemployment and lack of community resources.

Group members saw these three circles of deprivation as interacting and magnifying each other. For example, young people caused problems because they were bored due to the lack of leisure activities on the estate.

As a result, other vulnerable people were afraid to walk around the estate, with adverse health consequences such as stress, isolation and lack of exercise.

Poverty and unemployment
As already noted, residents saw poverty and unemployment as linked to poor health in a variety of ways, e.g. boredom, social isolation, financial stress and the inability to afford a healthy diet or leisure activities. Some group members expressed hostility towards what they saw as victim-blaming by the government and the media. What was rejected was not the health education message, but the failure to appreciate the social circumstances in which 'bad' health behaviours occurred.

> Another thing, they tell you on the telly, Social Security is supposed to be going to cut our money down because them who smokes are buying fags out of Social Security money. What else have we got? I mean, you can't have nowt else, so you might as well have that. (Woman carer)

Lack of community resources
The second circle of deprivation consisted of the lack of accessible social, leisure and shopping facilities. Residents felt doubly deprived because they could not afford private or public transport to get to the city centre but there were no facilities within easy walking distance. The main lacks mentioned included supermarkets with fresh, cheap vegetables, leisure centres providing opportunities for recreation, exercise, hobbies and social contacts, parks for young children and community policing.
Lack of social resources was thus seen squarely as a health issue.

> You can join ... you can form groups ... I mean, it isn't only health, as I said, it's health of the mind. It's helping you meeting people. (Unemployed man)

Shortcomings in health services
At a third level of deprivation, medical, community health and hospital services were criticized for failing to prevent or deal with health problems arising out of poverty/unemployment and lack of community resources. The present discussion will focus primarily on GP practices.
A few very positive statements were made by group members of all ages.

> The doctor who I go to, who I consider to be one of the best surgeries round here.... They're all treated like they were personal friends. (Elderly man)

However, the balance of comments was strongly negative. Criticisms centred on access, inappropriate kinds of services and unprofessional conduct by GPs.

One kind of access problem involved simply getting to the surgery (there were none on the estate). One unemployed single mother had suffered severe depression after the birth of her first baby and felt that she could not cope because the baby was constantly crying. When she made long journeys to her doctor's by bus, the baby would fall asleep and the doctor would dismiss her concerns, sending her home even more depressed. Minor injuries often caused problems because mothers had no-one to look after their other children while they made the lengthy journey to the nearest accident and emergency department.

Getting to see the doctor and obtaining home visits were recurring problems. Receptionists, the doctors' border guards, were sometimes criticized as unfriendly and unhelpful. Other group members had a perhaps more sophisticated view of receptionists as a buffer between doctor and patient. Several patients had found a way of manipulating the doctor through the receptionist, in order to get an appointment.

> Well, I phoned before, and asked for an appointment, I mean for my children, say, and she'll say 'Oh well, there's no appointment'. And I'll say 'Righto then, can you send the doctor out'. And she'll ... come back five minutes later, and you can go down. (Adult woman)

Group members felt that there were a number of services which they lacked and which GPs could not appropriately provide. There were frequent requests for counselling by insiders who had experienced life on the estate. Doctors, although sometimes seen as sympathetic and supportive, were generally considered to be unsuitable as counsellors, for various reasons including lack of time, gender and judgmental attitudes.

> Somebody who's not going to lecture you [needed to talk to] ... When I go to my doctor's, I always get a lecture. (Female carer)

Another unmet need was for local paramedical care provided by a nurse. This service could give minor first aid, advise whether a journey to the doctor was necessary and provide advocacy to get residents in to see the doctor, if necessary.

> You see, if you had ... somebody like a district nurse, somebody who was qualified, turned round, and said 'Well, I think you should see the doctor now' ... She'd have the authority as well, you see. (Adult woman)

A third important area of unmet need concerned sex education and sexual health. There was general agreement among young people and their parental generation that sex education was desperately needed but woefully inadequate. Young women did not want to discuss sexual matters with a male doctor and did not trust in their confidentiality.

Interviewer: Why wouldn't you use your doctor [for contraceptive advice]?

Because... I suppose it could still slip out to your parents, and you mightn't want your parents to know.

And, for a start, my doctor's a man, and so...

Mine is as well. (Girls aged 16–19)

Some group members produced 'horror stories' about doctors and community services. Three such stories are reproduced below. To put them in perspective, most group members had sufficient confidence in their doctors not to want to change even if one was offered on the estate, despite access problems. Nevertheless, incidents like those described below are disturbing.

Now, when my son had cancer ... he went to the doctor's that many times. The doctor turned round and says, 'Oh get out, always coming in with bad backs'. Now, do you call that a good doctor? I don't. (Adult woman)

They brought my dad from the home one night – one day. Never said they were bringing him, they just left him.... What does he do? Fell out of his wheelchair. You try to lift 15 stone. I had to lift him, with a next door neighbour, because I couldn't do it on my own. But to try to explain that to other people, they just don't listen, they don't want to know. (Female carer)

I know our X [suffering from anorexia], in her visit to ... the mind healer, or whatever he's called, he asked her if she wanted to be man more than she wanted to be woman. Did she get sexual pleasure out of vomiting? ... I used to think, like, punch me, how can you get sexual pleasure out of vomiting? (Mother of young children)

The last example illustrates the way in which a professional perspective, in this case a crude misconception of psychoanalysis, can lead to full-blown misunderstanding of the client's problem, with potentially disastrous results.

Community development and health

Each of the 16 groups felt that the most important thing that could be done to improve the health of residents of the estate was to provide a community/leisure/health centre. Different ideas were expressed about its detailed functions, but there was a striking consensus that the following features were desirable.

- Residents should have some 'ownership' of the centre, through participating in the management of its activities. A conventional health centre managed by doctors was not wanted.
- The centre should draw on 'alliances' between professionals and residents, whose experiential knowledge (e.g. about drug problems) and resources (e.g. the time of the unemployed) should be utilized.
- The centre should have a broad, holistic concept of health and take advantage of synergy between different spheres of activities, for example, offering health education advice to people drawn into the centre for leisure activities.
- The centre should have a community integration function, e.g. promoting positive contacts between different age groups.

Group members discussed a wide range of specific functions for the community/health centre. These included first aid, advice about the need to see a doctor, advocacy with doctors and receptionists, health and sex education, family planning and sexual health, counselling, welfare advice, leisure and fitness activities and encouraging social contacts. The quotation below illustrates some of these themes.

> We want a community centre built that accommodates everybody, all ages....
>
> So you're talking about a leisure centre?
>
> All in one....
>
> With a health centre built on, you know, like....
>
> If a young person on [the estate] went and speaks to old people, they think they're getting mugged. (Disabled men and women)

DISCUSSION

The HNP and the PS cannot be compared directly, since the populations which they represented were quite different. The HNP was conducted on the edge of a conurbation, in an area of extreme social disadvantage. The PS was carried out in small towns, villages and countryside, although one containing many areas with similarly high levels of unemployment and poverty. As discussed above, research initiated by GPs produced a better response rate than research started by community residents.

Despite methodological differences, there were some agreements between the results of the two projects. Access to doctors was mentioned frequently in the HNP, and was a problem for a substantial minority of patients in the PS, where it was associated with lower household social class. One reason for this may be that surgeries are less likely to be situated in socially deprived areas like that covered by the HNP.

Receptionists were seen as a barrier to access by participants in both projects, perhaps a reflection of their status as a buffer between doctors and patients, rather than their personal inadequacy. The HNP complemented the PS by illustrating the dynamics of the relationship between receptionist and patient, for example the manoeuvre of asking the doctor to make a home visit in order to get a speedier appointment at the surgery.

The 'pictures' of doctors and medical services associated with the two projects were very different. PS respondents were overwhelmingly positive about their doctors. For example, among the 31 respondents who were urban residents from unskilled manual social class backgrounds, over 90% felt that the doctor was good at listening and explaining, and over 80% considered him or her good at examining and prescribing.

Positive comments about GPs were made by respondents in the HNP, and most did not want to change their doctor. But negative, even virulent, comments were common. This difference may have a methodological explanation. The general questions in the PS may have evoked normative responses, reflecting the high esteem which doctors, in general, are still given in our culture. The HNP stimulated 'gossip mode', perhaps with a bias towards negative incidents which make better anecdotes. Neither project gives a 'true' picture of patient perceptions of GPs and each needs to be considered in relation to the method used to produce it.

Behind these methodological issues were differences of agenda. The PS was a consumer survey. Valuable information was generated about patients' evaluations of existing services. The FHSA's main conclusions for action were that money needed to be spent on improving the appearance of waiting rooms and that receptionists needed social skills training. Neither conclusion challenged doctors' roles by raising questions about the location of surgeries, access problems or the appropriateness of medical intervention.

Not one group member in the HNP mentioned the condition of the waiting room. Difficulties with the receptionist were seen as part of a wider problem of a user-unfriendly service. Participants in the HNP were more concerned with changing the nature of 'health' services, by gaining some degree of community control and by broadening their scope to include services such as first aid, medical advocacy, leisure/fitness, health education, counselling and welfare advice.

At the meeting which discussed the report, the FHSA did not support the proposal to develop a community/health/leisure centre in partnership with residents. Resource problems were not discussed, because of FHSA hostility to the idea in principle.

Members felt that there were legal objections to setting up a first aid station run by a nurse and to unemployed residents looking after children. They were concerned that the residents wanted to dispense with middle-class professionals and relieved when I assured them, using current jargon, that residents were seeking 'alliances'. Community participation was felt to be problematic, because activists were unrepresentative while representative people were apathetic. One member was indignant that boredom and lack of facilities were being used as 'excuses' for youthful criminal behaviour. As author of the report, I felt like a bad anthropologist who had identified too closely with the 'natives'.

In response to the report, the FHSA decided to consider a series of specific issues, including ability to register with a local GP, availability and delivery of dental and ophthalmic services and extending the role of the pharmacist. These issues, while undoubtedly important, appeared unrelated to those raised by residents. Their advantage for the FHSA may have been that they did not challenge professional control. Meanwhile, the women's community group that initiated the research is, at the time of writing, facing closure due to withdrawal of funding by the local community education service.

More generally, efforts are being made to tackle community problems like those shown up by the HNP in various ways. Locality planning by combined District Health Authorities and FHSA purchasers is attempting to profile the needs of localities and target services to meet those needs. The City Challenge initiative has directed substantial resources into improving poor city environments, including that on which the HNP was based. However, spending on inner city projects, including City Challenge, is now being cut sharply (*Guardian*, 5/3/94).

Although both initiatives are to be welcomed, their effectiveness needs to be closely monitored. They do not share control over resources with residents of localities, and they do not overcome the split between 'health' and 'social' care. Following the main HNP research discussed in this chapter an additional focus group was conducted with City Challenge representatives from the city in which the HNP took place. The seven participating representatives, from a possible maximum of 17, expressed disillusion with the early stages of City Challenge planning.

> And people have found that they're just up against another institution by a different name [City Challenge], with different people, but no more interested in what they really want. (City Challenge representative)

CHAPTER 5

Community maternity care

Joan E. Aarvold and Jean Davies

*The woman must be the focus of maternity care.
She should be able to feel in control of what is
happening to her and able to make decisions about
her care, based on her needs, having discussed
matters fully with the professionals involved.*
FIRST PRINCIPLE OF GOOD MATERNITY CARE. (DOH,
1993, P. 8)

INTRODUCTION

Looking at maternity care in a community framework raises some fundamental issues about the important role of birth within any society.

How it is managed and organized not only reflects the prevailing
ideology about fertility, but reinforces cultural identity. In Britain, health
care has become largely synonymous with medical care, which in turn
has become increasingly reliant on technology that plays a leading role in
the important 'rites of passage' at both ends of life. This technology,
because of its high cost, need for skilled operators and regular maintenance, is usually located in hospitals. Social and emotional aspects of birth
have become marginalized as maternity services have developed (Hare,
1972; Katz-Rothman, 1982; Jowitt, 1993). Having a medicalized, institutionalized birth fosters dependency on medicine at a crucial time and
reinforces medicalization throughout society.

Implicit in institutionalized birth is the belief that having a baby is a
'crisis' for the mother and child. Conversely, the traditional, community-
oriented philosophy is that childbirth is an inherently normal 'peak' experience. These diametrically opposed beliefs support very different types
of maternity service provision. Issues of power, control and status are
fundamental to the debate, and pervade both interprofessional and
professional–client relationships. The mother may be perceived by different professionals, at different stages, as patient, client or woman. The

former is dependent on the institution, whereas the latter signifies autonomy and a clear social role, independent of the institution. Pearson (Chapter 6), found that mothers also wanted a more reciprocal, autonomous relationship with health visitors in the community.

Community maternity care should be about recognizing and promoting the status of clients and, as the quote at the beginning of the chapter affirms, providing care to meet their needs. A pregnant woman and her family have psychological, emotional, social, financial and physical needs. Above all, maternity care should be women-centred.

The chapter is in two main parts. In the first, the authors discuss current maternity services in relation to the characteristics of community care outlined in Chapter 1. Some of the methodological problems faced by researchers in this field are then briefly examined. The second part of the chapter discusses two research projects. One was a controlled trial of the effects of enhanced community midwifery care in an economically disadvantaged community. The other was a survey of clients' opinions of note carrying and their information needs during antenatal care. The findings from both studies support the principle of a women-centred approach to maternity care.

The chapter concludes with a discussion of the paradox that certain groups of 'ill' people are being moved out of institutions into the community, while the maternally 'well' are generally institutionalized.

BACKGROUND

Definitions and development

Two themes recur in the critical literature about maternity services in the UK. One is that the perceived needs of women and service provision are often not confluent (Graham, 1978; Inch, 1981; Oakley, 1984; Garcia, Kilpatrick and Richards, 1990). The other is that service development is based on medical orthodoxy (Campbell and Macfarlane, 1987; Tew, 1990).

A series of government reports over the last 30 years have been instrumental in shaping policy (MOH, 1959, 1970; House of Commons Social Services Committee, 1980). Much of the evidence on which these reports were based came from medical advisers who believed that birth outside hospital was potentially dangerous. In contrast, midwives' main remit is to care for healthy women, whose pregnancies should be treated as normal. The latest government report (DOH, 1993) signifies a radical change in this direction. Its first principle, that women must be the focus of care, is indicative of the bizarre fact that birth had become more medically than socially focused.

Maternity care, unlike most other community health care provision, has clear boundaries. A woman usually enters the system, via the gatekeeper GP, at a self-selected stage in her pregnancy, most commonly during the first three months. Very few women receive no antenatal care, although there are class and age differences in attendance rates (Rantakallio, 1979; O'Brien and Smith, 1981). The GP will usually refer the woman to a large obstetric unit where her antenatal visits are organized according to criteria based on practices established in the 1920s (MOH, 1929). The average number of antenatal visits has gone up from 8.1 per woman in 1950 to 10.4 in 1978 (Oakley, 1982). Increasing the number of antenatal clinic visits has not been found to improve outcomes for all women, but this medically determined pattern of care persists (Enkin and Chalmers, 1982).

Antenatal care in Britain may be 'shared' with the woman's GP, and a midwife may preside over all or some of the visits. Sharing, however, refers to care being divided between the GP and the hospital, not to communicating with the pregnant woman. A woman may opt to have all of her antenatal care at the hospital, or may be advised to do so for medical reasons.

In labour, and for delivery, a woman is cared for by a midwife, but a doctor is usually involved at some point. Although the pattern of care varies in different localities, most births take place in Britain within a structure that is obstetrically ordained and organized. Following the birth, care for the mother and baby is mostly carried out by midwives, both in the hospital and at home.

The Local Government Act of 1974 transferred midwives from local authority to health authority control and was pivotal in the transition from home to hospital delivery. Obstetric consultant posts continued to rise while the number of community midwives fell (Campbell and Macfarlane, 1987). With the closure of most small maternity units and lack of support for home births, choice for users of maternity services has been limited (Davies, 1982).

Characteristics of community maternity care

In Chapter 1, community health care was differentiated from purely medical care in terms of the following characteristics.

- It is about behaviour, psychology, social lifestyle and economic consequences of health issues.
- It is critical of institutionalized care.
- It utilizes community resources.

In terms of these three characteristics, maternity services in Britain fall short of providing community health care.

Holistic care

Having a baby affects not just a woman's physical condition, but also her social, interpersonal and psychological state (Kitzinger, 1978; Oakley, 1985). Becoming a parent within our social structure and giving birth have somehow become separated. The medicalized maternity service takes little account of a woman's expectations of parenthood and ability to mother her baby, and even less account of the father's new role (Lomas, 1964; Lewis, 1986). Although some of a woman's care may be delivered 'in the community', i.e. outside hospital, this care is given under the GP's authority and generally follows the medical model.

A woman can be made to feel anxious during her pregnancy through her contact with the service. A date of delivery, predicted by scan, may conflict with her own estimated length of pregnancy. She may be told that her weight gain is either too much or too little, that the size of the uterus is not quite right or that her blood glucose level is slightly raised. This preoccupation with physical measurement deflects from the social and emotional changes taking place during pregnancy. Anxiety itself affects not only a woman's labour and birth, but also her mothering experiences (Jowitt, 1993).

Many pregnant women have real concerns about welfare benefits and lifestyle issues (Aarvold, 1989). They also want information about their pregnancy and baby care and continually seek reassurance (Artells, 1988). In the past, this reassurance would have come from within the community, but is now sought from a health service which is seldom equipped to give it. When a woman decides that other things in her life take precedence over attending for an antenatal appointment, her behaviour is considered irrational and professionals label her as a defaulter (Graham, 1978). Even in 'at risk' pregnancies, where there is physical cause for concern, being monitored outside hospital has been found to lower anxiety levels and to have clear benefits for the woman and her family (Middlemiss *et al.*, 1989).

The birth environment itself also appears to play a crucial role in a woman's sense of control and subsequent self-esteem. Hodnett (1989) found that women who chose to have their babies at home enjoyed greater continuity of care, lower noise and light levels and a greater sense of freedom and comfort. As a result, they had significantly higher levels of perceived control than women delivering in hospital.

Before the changes in the 1970s from local authority to medical control discussed above, midwives were known in the community. Their roles were recognized by the families they visited. Subsequently, social and psychological concerns became subordinate to matters of medicine and pathology.

Institutional versus *women-centred care*

The series of reports mentioned earlier, on which the present maternity service is based, were compiled mostly by medical men and claimed that all births should be conducted within the safety of the hospital environment. This belief was probably the result of their experiences of home births, to which they would only be called if there was an emergency. Discussions of home births often produce anecdotal tales of terror. Doctors' experiences of normal neighbourhood birthing tend to be limited.

Falling perinatal and maternal mortality rates in developed countries have coincided with increasing hospitalization of births. The medical establishment has propagated the belief that the latter has 'caused' the former. Tew (1990) has brought together evidence which supports the alternative hypothesis that increased 'safety' in childbirth is primarily the result of raised living and nutritional standards.

Hospitalization of births leads to institutional, bureaucratic, rather than user-centred, care. Stafford (1993), through her role as Director of Consumer Affairs, Leeds FHSA, has developed a set of quality indicators for the provision of local maternity services which are based on user as well as professional views. Women felt that higher priority needed to be given to privacy, dignity, cultural awareness, appropriateness of information and non-judgemental advice on diet, smoking and alcohol.

The institutional, medical model which prevails has also had an important influence on the training of midwives. Until very recently, most entrants into midwifery training were qualified nurses. Since 1990 several colleges and universities have offered 'direct entry', three year courses leading to registration. These programmes are attracting small numbers of women who have had other life experiences outside school and hold a more social view of maternity care. However, the majority of practising midwives are, and for some time will continue to be, products of a medical, nurse-training model, oriented to caring for sick people. It is not difficult, within this model, to convince those who had assumed birth to be a normal physiological event that it is inherently pathological. Student midwives are given community experience. They visit mothers at home and in community clinics but will seldom see antenatal, perinatal and postnatal care delivered entirely by midwives outside the medical structure.

Utilizing community resources

Government funding has been directed towards supporting hospital births and away from facilitating family participation. Grants given to mothers having home confinements were phased out in the late 1960s.

Paternity leave is currently not supported. Paid maternity leave is limited. The home help service, once available to new mothers, is now virtually non-existent. The maternity grant, previously awarded to all pregnant women, has been abolished. The only available grant is means-tested. However, it is possible for GPs to be paid for each pregnancy and they can receive more than the means-tested woman.

Holland, in contrast to the UK, has maintained a system organized around home birth and support for the family. Midwifery is financed and organized as an autonomous profession (van Teijlingen and McCaffery, 1987). Dutch political commitment to the family is reflected in the provision of trained home helps for all new mothers during the crucial early days of mothering.

Maternity services in the UK are currently based on a philosophy of hospital/crisis, rather than community/peak. Dependency on services is stimulated by strict surveillance of pregnancy and medicalized control over the birth. The family is then left to get on with parenting. Midwives, who were more involved with the woman and her family, have had their role undermined by relocation into the hospital.

Fathers are also affected by hospitalization, often having to go home to an empty house, or to manage visiting while coping with other children. Birth is a peak experience which can have an enormous effect on a partnership. The concession to 'allow' fathers to be in hospital for the birth does not get over the fact that at a time of heightened emotion there is separation. It is akin to having two red hot pieces of metal that need to be welded together kept separate until they have cooled down.

Adequate and appropriate preparation for the role of parent should be promoted by a system which places the family in a position of responsibility, competence and high status. Hospital confinements themselves need not thwart these objectives, but the current system does, because the institution dominates.

Before birth was medicalized, grandmothers, neighbours, siblings and fathers played their part. Now the medical gaze rests predominantly on the woman, isolated from her family. Maternity care in the UK appears to be lagging historically behind other forms of care, e.g. for the mentally ill, where there have been shifts towards an orientation to the whole person.

Far from using the resources of the family and the community, women are admitted to hospital, separated from their communities, to await their babies' births. This practice denies communities the culturally cohesive event of birth. It is beginning to be considered as a possible contributing factor to the breakdown of family structures.

A model for community maternity care

The present medicalized system of maternity care is bound up with power structures in which consultants (mostly male) dominate users (female) and midwives (mostly female). Where midwives are autonomous care givers, as in Holland, women giving birth enjoy high status and full participation in care. Figure 5.1 illustrates the potential progression from a traditional, institutional model of care to a partnership, community model.

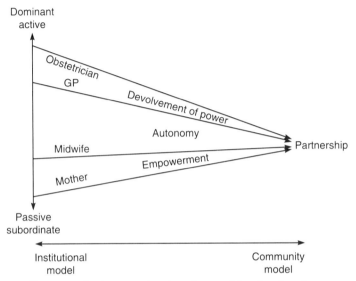

Figure 5.1   Framework of power structure for models of maternity care.

To enable those in subordinate positions to move towards a more equal status, as shown in the figure above, those occupying dominant positions will have to relinquish some of their power. Partnership in care requires not only a change in power distribution, but also a desire on the part of the subordinate members for more autonomy. Some midwives have come to accept a subservient role which is consistent with women's experiences generally (Barclay, 1986). The general public will also need re-educating. The belief that birth can only be seen to be normal in retrospect, and requires medical surveillance, has become pervasive in the western world. The Changing Childbirth Report (DOH, 1993) recommends that at least 30% of women should have the midwife as their lead professional. This displacement of the obstetrician will not only enable a midwife to use her skills to the full but, together with a shift of care away from the hospital outlined in the report, will lead to women themselves playing a greater part in their own care.

User perspectives

Research into user perspectives on maternity services has taken the form of either opinion surveys (O'Brien and Smith, 1981; Boyd and Sellers,

1982; Association of Community Health Councils for England and Wales, 1987; Amoss, Jones and Martin, 1988; Which, 1989; Small, Lumley and Brown, 1992) or evaluations of new approaches to service delivery (Flint and Poulengeris, 1987; Middlemiss *et al.*, 1989; Williams *et al.*, 1989). As pointed out in Chapter 2, interpretation of consumer satisfaction surveys is problematic (Jacoby and Cartwright, 1990; McIver, 1992). Questions tend to be constructed around health service providers' ideas of what is important for patients. Typically, surveys are then copied from one authority to another, under the assumption that, because certain questions have been asked, they must be crucial ones. Other drawbacks relate to sensitivity of the survey tool, language barriers and underestimation of the resources needed for complete analysis and report writing. Many are left to gather dust on shelves.

Comparative studies between midwifery-led community provision, with a large proportion of births occurring outside hospital, and the present obstetrically based, hospitalized system are not possible. Similarly, asking women their opinion of a community midwifery service is rather meaningless when they have no experience on which to base an answer.

Schemes based on a midwifery-led approach have been initiated in the UK and abroad. Sakala (1989) discusses an independent midwifery service developed in Massachusetts USA for low income groups. In this service, midwives are autonomous practitioners who decide whether to refer to a consultant. Although the majority of births take place in hospital, the aim is to provide care that is accessible, dignifying, health-promoting and empowering. The project has achieved better rates of low birth weight, neonatal mortality and breast feeding than were found in the wider service area. However, the users of this service could not afford care managed by physicians. It is possible that this small-scale scheme was only tolerated because it did not involve financial loss to the medical profession.

Another example of women-centred, midwifery-led service in the UK was the 'Know your midwife' scheme (Flint and Poulengeris, 1987). This scheme operated within the hospital environment, but enabled midwives to give continuity of care to women. Although high levels of satisfaction were expressed by mothers and midwives and outcomes were favourable, the scheme was not consolidated following evaluation. Resources can always be found, it appears, for new technology, but seldom for structural changes. However, the scheme has influenced the political climate and the development of maternity services.

The research ethos

The prevailing research ethos largely reinforces the medicalization of birth. Research has been dominated by a 'scientific' paradigm which emphasizes quantification and linear reductionism. Topic selection, theoretical analysis and methodology tend to reflect men's experiences, ideas and needs. Women appear most often as objects of enquiry. Such research neither illuminates nor helps to alleviate women's inferior status. Midwives have lacked the confidence to develop their own research tradition (McCool and McCool, 1989; Hicks, 1992). However, the midwifery profession is in an excellent position to incorporate new feminist approaches (Daley, 1993) which focus on women's experiences and demonstrate a concern for values.

Implementation of successful, innovative practices into mainstream care will depend on the relative power of the various interest groups. Success may, to the manager, be measured in cost-effective terms. To the obstetrician, it may be measured in lower perinatal mortality rates (PNMRs). To the midwife, it may mean more job satisfaction, through being able to provide continuity of care. And, to the woman recipient, it may be measured in terms of more control over and satisfaction with her birthing experience. The 'effectiveness' of community midwifery cannot be assessed by a single measure. The definition of effectiveness is a political issue.

THE COMMUNITY MIDWIFERY CARE PROJECT

Introduction

The Newcastle Community Midwifery Care Project was set up in 1983. A full time researcher was employed to evaluate the initiative which ran for three years (Evans, 1987). Four midwives worked in two areas of the city with high rates of economic deprivation and unemployment. The aims of the study were:

- to provide enhanced support by midwives to mothers in their own homes in areas with a high prevalence of risk factors;
- to assess the effects of the intervention on outcome, consumer satisfaction and relationships between hospital and community services.

Each woman was allocated a named midwife, who provided continuous care. The midwife visited the mother at home at least four times antenatally, offering locally based parentcraft classes, and visited her in hospital and postnatally up to the 28th day. As the midwives worked in the neighbourhood, their presence became accepted. Pregnancies were often 'reported' to the midwives long before a mother would have normally visited her GP.

Methodology

Four evaluation methods were used: client, staff and case note surveys and a time budget study.

The client survey

The intervention group consisted of 263 women who 'booked' from the two study areas between October 1984 and 1985. The control group consisted of 208 women who came from comparable areas elsewhere in the city. Women from the study and control groups were matched for age, parity, social class, marital status, place of delivery and type of ante-natal care. The women were interviewed twice, antenatally (during their last trimester) and postnatally (at about six weeks). There were 12 miscarriages and 12 house moves in the intervention group, leaving a total of 239 participants. The response rates were, for the intervention group, 84% antenatal and 75% postnatal and for the control group, 87% antenatal and 88% postnatal. A total of 812 interviews were completed.

The interviews, undertaken by the project researcher (Francis Evans), used open-ended questions which were recorded in full and postcoded. The topics included experience of service and lifestyle issues.

Case note survey

The case notes of the intervention group were compared with those of two additional control groups: firstly a retrospective control group consisting of all the women in the intervention areas who delivered the year before the study (1982/3); and secondly a matched control group selected in the same way as outlined above. In all, 862 case notes were reviewed, and information was collected postnatally about the outcome of pregnancy and clinical management.

Staff survey

A variety of professionals were interviewed, including the four Project midwives, locally based GPs and health visitors, the consultant obstetricians, the hospital antenatal sister, the Director and Assistant Director of Midwifery, the Senior Midwifery Tutor and all the other community midwives within the health authority. The Project mothers were registered with 27 different GP practices, only five worked within the Project area. A written enquiry to all 27 practices yielded a practice response rate of 59% ($n = 16$).

Time budget study

The four Project midwives and nine midwives working in the control areas completed a detailed account of a full working week.

Results

The client survey

Women in the intervention group were significantly more satisfied with the service than those in the matched control group (Evans, 1987). Antenatally, 77% of 198 'cases' said that they were very satisfied, compared with 35% of 184 controls. Postnatally, 77% of cases were very satisfied, compared with 55% of controls.

Recorded comments fill out the reasons mothers gave for satisfaction with the Community Midwifery Project.

> I was very satisfied. It is an important time in your life. You want to feel important, and the midwives I saw did that for me, they made me feel really important.

There was dissatisfaction about many environmental issues. In the case group, 78% of women indicated that their housing provision caused major problems and anxiety. Burglary, vandalism, low income/debt and dogs were frequently cited concerns. Medical surveillance was not considered a priority need by these families.

Case notes

The case note survey showed that there were also clinical benefits. The numbers were too small for the perinatal mortality rates to be affected, but there was evidence that the enhanced care reduced the incidence of premature births.

In the intervention group, 6% ($n = 14$) of all mothers had preterm deliveries, compared with 11% ($n = 23$) in the retrospective control group. Among cases, 21% ($n = 29$) of women who had had a previous low birth weight baby (< 2500 g) had another at the end of the study pregnancy, compared with 46% ($n = 96$) among controls. There was a smaller difference among women who had not had a previous low birth weight baby. Prematurity and low birth weight are the two main contributing factors in PNMRs. Although the numbers involved were small, the Project had an impact on these two outcomes.

The staff survey

The staff survey showed that Project midwives felt that it enabled them to improve relationships with their clients.

> You are able to give continuity of care. In hospital it is all interruptions.... With this, you go and see somebody, and do everything that she needs. And you finish with her before you move on to the next.

The Project midwives felt that relationships between community midwives and those working in the hospital had improved. There was more contact and sharing of information about some of the women, particularly those who were a cause for concern. Social problems that were not necessarily evident in a hospital setting were more likely to be recognized in the antenatal care of individual women. Being community based, the midwives were frequently hailed in the street, and given information about problems relating to their clients. In this way, the midwives were able to play a role in challenging the effects of socioeconomic disadvantage, providing enhanced support and education.

Most of the other professionals working in the community with the same group of women welcomed the Project as benefiting the women. The health visitors felt that liaison between them and the Project midwives was improved, partly because the midwives were geographically rather than GP based. Health visitors reported that enhanced confidence in the Project mothers made them more willing users of child health services. However, GPs at one of the four practices in the area expressed a negative view, that the Project interfered with their team approach.

Some members of the wider medical and midwifery communities were critical. Their reactions can be summarized as follows.

- If you enhance care – of course it will be better.
- Demonstrating that the controls were less satisfied implied that non-Project midwives were giving a poor service.

Time budget study

The time study showed that all community midwives, both Project and those working in the rest of the city, worked considerably longer than their contracted hours.

Implications of the project

This work was carried out with a client group who continue to have disproportionately high PNMRs. Those involved in the project felt that the evaluation had proved its usefulness in improving both user satisfaction and clinical outcomes, and that it should be extended. However, the Project was not consolidated.

The dismissal of some the findings, and of a model of care which would reduce medical control over midwives, is an illustration of medical power within the maternity services in the area where the study took place. In some other parts of Britain, real attempts have been made to introduce and support a more community oriented service. The Sighthill Community Antenatal Care Scheme (McKee, 1984) is favourably reported.

Women are seen less often, for a well defined purpose, by midwives in community-based clinics. Care is flexible and not duplicated in unnecessary hospital visits.

ANTENATAL INFORMATION SURVEY

Introduction

This study was initiated and carried out in 1988 by lay members of the local Maternity Services Liaison Committee (MSLC) with support from the Community Health Council (CHC). Without the support of the CHC, the lay members might not have succeeded in getting the research proposal approved by the medical members of the MSLC.

The survey was undertaken in Newcastle's two maternity hospitals to evaluate a new system of note carrying, and to discover what mothers felt about the information available to them during their antenatal care.

Note carrying by clients is a contentious issue. Many reasons can be found for keeping notes in the hospital. The most usual ones given are that patients might lose them or be made anxious by reading them. Where maternity clients have been entrusted with their notes, neither problem has arisen (Lovell *et al.*, 1986; Elbourne *et al.*, 1987).

In Newcastle it was decided that clients could not be allowed to hold their complete case notes. Instead a compromise solution was tried out. For women receiving shared care only, the current maternity notes were to be photocopied, with one copy kept by the mother. Client opinion of the 'new' system was sought after it had been in operation for two years. At the same time, the opportunity to assess client satisfaction with antenatal information was taken.

Methodology

Sample characteristics

All women in the third trimester of pregnancy attending both units during a one-week period were invited to participate in the study. Liaison workers from ethnic minority groups were informed of the survey and were able to encourage non-English-speaking women to participate. Over 90% of women attending during the study week participated in the survey. 204 questionnaires were returned, about half from each unit. This represents 28% of the total population. It cannot, therefore, be assumed that the sample was representative.

Within this sample, 77% ($n = 157$) of women were receiving shared care whilst the remaining 23% ($n = 47$) attended the hospital for all their antenatal checks.

Methods

The data were obtained by questionnaire only. The design of the questionnaire involved consultation with midwives, doctors and lay people, and consideration of previously validated survey work of this nature (Elbourne *et al.*, 1987). A pilot study (45 questionnaires) enabled the researchers to test the willingness of the women to participate, to see whether or not the exercise was in any way intrusive to the running of the clinic, and to modify the presentation.

The questionnaire was a mixture of 15 open and closed questions. The latter referred to age, postcode, parity, type of care, sources of information and aspects of note carrying. Questions pertaining to information and ideas for improvement were given a five-point rating scale. Open comments were invited in two places, relating to information received and recommendations for improvements.

Results

Note keeping

The number of women who reported having a photocopy of their notes (179) was greater than the number having shared care (157), suggesting that some consultants were involving hospital-only patients in the scheme. Of the 179 women who received a photocopy, 88% (158) said they always read it. However, only 32% (57) of those reading their notes said they always understood them. The main reasons given for misunderstanding were problems with medical words and handwriting.

Of the women who had a photocopy, 92% (164) said they would want a copy for a subsequent pregnancy and 92% (23) of those who had no written record said they would prefer to have one. Women who carried their notes were asked to indicate advantages and disadvantages. Women felt that having their own notes improved their understanding and control of the pregnancy and enhanced their ability to communicate with professionals. Only 4% (2) felt that they were worrying to read.

Information giving

Current medical information (scans, routine tests) was rated most favourably, but the majority did not rate information on wider aspects of pregnancy (e.g. diet, smoking, alcohol consumption, maternity benefits) as good. Those receiving shared care were more likely to rate information as good than those receiving hospital care only. Suggestions for improving communication included mothers reading their own notes, more time with doctors and midwives and a glossary of medical terms.

Implications

Most respondents valued being given written information about their pregnancies. Despite problems over legibility and understanding, women who carried their own notes felt more involved in their pregnancies. The results support the Changing Childbirth (DOH, 1993, p. 13) recommendation that women should carry their own case notes if they wish. However, the shared care differed from the hospital-only group in other aspects of their treatment, as well as note keeping, and are likely to have differed in other ways associated with their selection for a particular type of care.

Levels of satisfaction with information about wider aspects of pregnancy were low, particularly among women who were being cared for solely by the hospital. It became apparent during the pilot study that some women did not realize that hospital midwives were able to answer questions.

It should be of great concern that women themselves are not satisfied with the information they receive about the wider aspects of having a baby, for example about the effects of lifestyle on the baby's health and about financial matters. The shortcomings which the mothers identified arise from a maternity service which focuses on biological processes and fails to tackle the social context of birth, even in areas which affect the medical outcome of pregnancy directly, e.g. alcohol and smoking.

DISCUSSION

Maternity services must be readily accessible to all women. They should be sensitive to the needs of the local population and based primarily in the community.

SECOND PRINCIPLE OF GOOD MATERNITY CARE.
(DOH, 1993, P. 8)

Childbearing women are the subject matter of one of the most formidable disciplines in medicine. Paradoxically, while disadvantaged groups such as the elderly and the mentally ill are being moved out of institutional care, sometimes, arguably, to their disadvantage or that of their families, most pregnant women who could be cared for in the community by midwives are institutionalized, and placed under the surveillance of obstetricians.

Maternity provision does not appear to have responded to the findings of numerous consumer satisfaction surveys over the last 15 years, referenced in the Introduction to this chapter, particularly in relation to antenatal care. Problematic areas consistently referred to include inadequate information, lack of continuity of care, failure to meet individual needs and excessive waiting times. Examples of women-centred, midwifery-led care, like the Community Midwifery Care Project discussed in this chapter, are not only popular with mothers and midwives but are clinically beneficial (Oakley, 1985). Yet they are not being widely promoted or extended, even though midwives are cheaper to train and employ than doctors and are more able to provide holistic care.

Consumer opinion surveys may appease pressure groups who need keeping at bay, but have not led to real change. Despite a small but growing number of women, midwives and doctors who would like to see a women-centred, midwifery-led, community-based service, resources are not as yet being directed to this aim.

Consumer criticisms of the information they receive indicate that women's needs are not always addressed or met. Women are concerned about family, lifestyle and role change as well as the medical aspects of pregnancy. Community midwives are in an excellent position to be able to address the needs of pregnant and new mothers, particularly those who figure disproportionately in the PNMR tables. An overly medical service orientation is preventing midwives from developing this wider role.

The consultants involved with the Project did not feel it had affected the clinical management of pregnancy. They made very little use of the additional midwifery resources, retaining traditional hospital clinic visiting practices, despite the care available to mothers in the community. In a response to The Changing Childbirth Report (DOH, 1993), local obstetricians stated: 'The high standards achieved in the hospital midwifery service within the City must be sustained and not sacrificed in the pursuit of community midwifery *per se'*. (Division of Obstetrics and Gynaecology Newcastle HA, Point 6, p. 2, 1993). Resistance to change may be based on lack of trust, ignorance of other forms of care or a desire to remain in control of maternity services.

Powerful traditions in maternity care are now being challenged, and there is a new emphasis on women-centred community care (House of Commons Health Committee, 1992; DOH, 1993). To move towards the community model advocated in this chapter demands a major political shift, involving change in the attitudes of senior obstetricians, re-education of the public, and requiring more confident midwives. It is now proposed (DOH, 1993) that midwives become the prime carers for pregnant women, who will have direct access to them in the community. This radical proposal for service provision will require major changes in role relationships between doctors and midwives.

Women are to be given real choice over the place of birth, with support for birth at home for those who wish it. Midwives should have access to hospital beds for their clients, where women can have holistic care should they prefer this environment. Medical resistance to birth outside hospital has always been very strong. However, it is imperative that the debate does not become polarized and focus simply on the merits of home versus hospital. The real debate should be about power and control within the whole service.

CHAPTER 6

Client views of health visiting

Pauline Pearson

INTRODUCTION

In this chapter a qualitative study, examining the ways in which mothers with very young children viewed the health visiting service, is discussed in the context of current debates about the role of health visitors. Methodological issues of access, sampling, ethics and longitudinal design are also considered.

Data from the study are used to illustrate the emergent theory. Clients' views of health and health visitors' roles alter over time, and relationships between client and health visitor perceptions also shift. These shifts can be seen in the development of the parent, the child and the health visitor/client relationship. Although studies of client perspectives can help practitioners to focus and reprioritize their work, the 'new' consumers of services are the purchasers, rather than the clients. When health is defined as a product, lay people's agendas may fall by the wayside.

BACKGROUND

Health visiting – the context

Health visiting in the United Kingdom has had a long and proud history, starting in the mid-19th century. Originating in sanitary inspection and public health, health visitors are now nurses trained to work in health promotion with adults, children and communities. Over the past 25 years, a major part of health visitors' work has been with families and children, screening for disease and developmental delay and offering advice and support with parenting. About 70% of visits by health visitors fall into this category (Clark, 1973; Dunnell and Dobbs, 1982).

Work with elderly people has also formed an important health promotion focus for health visitors. However, there has been an underlying debate about other appropriate roles for the profession, and the cartoon depicting one elderly lady saying to another 'the health visitor – is that the woman who calls every week to explain her role?' has more than a grain of truth in it. Health visitors are involved in 'community development' work related to health, with an underlying philosophy of 'empowerment'. There is also increasing debate about health visitors' public health role (Symonds, 1993). Because of the direction of the research described in this chapter, the health visitor's role other than with parents with young children will not be discussed further.

Health visitors' work has always been less easy to quantify than that of 'hands on' nurses (Clark, 1981). The public, despite always being the primary 'client' of health visitors, has seemed to have a very limited understanding of the role. In part this has been because of changes, ill understood – the health visitor as 'the woman from the welfare' taking on a wider role. In part, it has also been because the profession itself has been unclear. A number of documents (Council for the Education and Training of Health Visitors, 1977; Health Visitors Association, 1981; Royal College of Nursing, 1983) have been published by the profession, attempting to clarify what it is, what it should be doing, and where it should be going. As one such document had it, *Whither Health Visiting?* (Goodwin 1982).

One central and enduring document (Council for the Education and Training of Health Visitors, 1977) identified four principles of health visiting. Twinn and Cowley (1992) suggest that these remain a cornerstone of current practice. They are:

- searching out health needs;
- stimulating awareness of health needs;
- influencing policies affecting health;
- facilitating health-enhancing activities.

It is, however, open to debate how far individual health visitors actually undertake these roles and how far, in practice, they have a narrower focus on specific areas, such as developmental surveillance.

The above principles contain important assumptions, which may or may not be shared by clients. Most importantly, they assume that health is a clearly defined concept. In health visitor education, considerable time is spent in discussing models of health and on internalizing a broad-based operational concept of health (Cowley, 1991; Dingwall, 1977). But clients' own understanding of health is rarely considered.

Cornwell (1984) argued that methods of researching concepts of health must permit people to draw on personal and relatively concrete experiences rather than 'public' generalities. Lay people and professionals frequently construct health as the converse of illness, thus adopting a medical model (see Chapter 1). However, Cornwell (1984, p. 195) found that health services for children appear to be understood in a different way to those for adults, largely because health is seen as essentially normal for children. In consequence, health care relates to 'common sense' decisions about health, 'health problems which are not illness' and 'normal illness' (p. 195). Acute adult care relates, more often, to 'serious illness'. Cornwell's work illustrates relationships between perceptions of health and perceptions of services.

A further assumption of the principles of health visiting, outlined above, is that health needs can be clearly defined. But health needs, like health, can be construed in many ways by different individuals or agencies. The health need identified by the purchasing authority may not equate with that seen by the provider unit, the individual professional practitioner or the service user, as argued in Chapter 1. While the client may see an urgent need for, say, treatment for a speech problem for her daughter, the health visitor may identify, for example, a need for support for the parents. The provider unit may see a limited need for speech therapy, based on the assessed problem, and fail to identify any parental support need, particularly if staff are limited. The purchaser may feel that speech problems in this age group are less significant than some other needs, and so deprioritize them.

Health visitors often see themselves as facilitating clients' efforts to enhance their own health or, in current jargon, 'empowering' clients. Health professionals often use these terms loosely with little thought of the requirement to create a new balance, to share power over information and choice. This issue arises in most of the chapters in this volume, particularly Chapter 5. The process of professionalization has been described as a process of gaining power through control of knowledge (Johnson, 1972). Health visitors may feel that empowerment threatens their power base. At the same time, empowerment gives lay people greater self-esteem, resources and choice. This is a crucial element of the new 'consumer-driven' NHS in theory, but more difficult to achieve in practice, perhaps because it is less acceptable to professionals.

Another assumption, implicit in the four principles outlined above, is that health-enhancing activities can be well defined and understood. In reality, health visitors must question the evidence presented to them, by journals, official documents and free leaflets, much of which is partisan (e.g. health promotion leaflets put out by the Butter Council and various margarine manufacturers) or based on very limited material. The knowledge on which some of the professionals' power is based is, in practice, a shaky edifice. This is highlighted, for many parents, when they note that advice about second and subsequent children, for example, about sleeping position or contraindications to immunization, conflicts with what they were told last time around.

Parental perspectives on health visiting

Becoming a parent, particularly for the first time, usually involves a major life transition. Clulow (1982) discusses the alterations which occur in the relationship between the new parents as they incorporate a third party. It is not surprising, therefore, that the content of discussions with health visitors ranges more widely than childcare issues, including adult diet, marital disharmony and mental illness (Clark, 1973). Oakley (1981a, p. 308) describes the new parent as travelling 'in a foreign country', and finding that communication of their experiences 'is hindered by the gap between mother and expert'. She suggests that experts too rarely see experience as any sort of qualification, despite its important role in empirical testing of theory.

Roche and Stacey (1986) list 35 papers concerned with parental attitudes towards child health services. Mayall and Grossmith (1985) found that mothers' satisfaction with health visitors was generally high, but that mothers from social classes IV and V were less satisfied, perhaps because they were 'more vulnerable to the inspecting side of the health visitor' (Mayall, 1986, p. 165).

Graham (1979), Buswell (1980) and Field *et al.* (1982) all describe a degree of parental dissatisfaction with child health service provision. Field *et al.* (1982) classified the responses of 60% of mothers about their health visitors as positive, 20% as hostile and 20% as indifferent. Many mothers expressed criticisms of child health clinics, feeling that staff were too busy, there was too much queuing and a lack of privacy. Buswell (1980), in a qualitative, longitudinal study of the first year of life, found that a drop in clinic attendance occurred at about six months. Mothers cited the conflicting advice they received as a reason for this. Buswell notes that mothers turned more to their lay referral network (relatives and friends) for advice at this stage.

Orr (1980), in her study of health visiting, suggested four principal causes of problems of service delivery: fragmentation, e.g. between health clinics and GPs, leading to conflicting advice; inaccessibility, geographical or cultural; discontinuity, e.g. due to personnel changes; and unaccountability. It remains to be seen how far the 1990 health service reforms will improve the situation.

METHODOLOGY

Introduction

In the early 1980s, I was working with community groups consisting mainly of mothers in an inner city area of Newcastle. They gradually gained confidence in sharing their views of my colleagues and the services of which we were part. I became aware that I knew very little about how clients viewed health visiting. It seemed worthwhile to explore clients' views more systematically. Indeed, if one was to effectively search out health needs and facilitate people in health enhancing activities, a clear understanding of client perspectives was essential. At the same time, the rise of the early phase of consumerism in the NHS, following the Griffiths Report on Health Service Management (Griffiths, 1983), made client perspectives an important agenda item for managers as well as the profession. The study described in this chapter was funded by a Research Studentship from Newcastle Health Authority.

The study's aims were:

- to explore the process by which members of a client group identify and interpret their health needs;
- to examine the process by which members of a client group develop perceptions of health visiting services;
- to compare the perspectives of clients and health visitors;
- to make comparisons between the perceptions of clients from priority areas (relatively deprived) and non-priority areas (relatively affluent).

The research utilized a symbolic interactionist perspective, focusing on the meanings attached to health and to health visiting by clients. It was carried out in two phases. In Phase One, after piloting with a group, semi-structured interviews were conducted, in 1984, with a random sample of 41 parents of children aged between six and 12 months, living in priority and non-priority areas. About half the sample completed a free text diary focusing on the child's health status and contacts with health professionals for one week.

In Phase Two, which looked at processes, 19 primiparous mothers were interviewed on three occasions over a 10-month period during 1986–7. Interviewing commenced antenatally and finished when their child was around eight months old. Interviews were carried out with 10 of the mothers' health visitors in parallel, within two weeks of each parent interview.

The sample

Access and gatekeeping

Access to the research site is rarely discussed in textbooks. For the social scientist approaching an alien environment, it may be difficult even to find out who the gatekeepers are. In a complex organization like the NHS, there are gatekeepers at many levels. Cormack (1992) described some of the difficulties of entry to NHS sites and staff, for example, deciding upon the appropriate level, management or staff, at which to commence access.

For a health professional, these difficulties can be compounded by one's own place within the organization. For this study, in Phase One, I obtained permission to utilize a sample taken from the Child Health Computer (a District-wide system collecting immunization and surveillance data on all children) through the District Ethical Committee. At the time this Committee normally required a (medical) consultant's signature on the lengthy application form, but were content in this case with the cooperation of the Unit management, the support of local GPs and appropriate academic supervision.

At Phase Two, access was required to antenatal mothers. Again the Ethical Committee had to be negotiated, but this time the form included the support of the consultant, who was willing to provide access to 'his' patients. Once booked into a hospital, these women, still resident in the community and essentially well, had become medicalized as 'patients' (see Chapter 5). The medical 'ownership' of patients means, particularly in community settings, that people who in all other respects are healthy adults are normally approached (whether they realize it or not) to take part in health research via medical gatekeepers. Society's appropriate concern with intrusive, damaging or otherwise unethical research leads to a perceived need for a trustworthy arbiter. Doctors are viewed as a reliable judge in these matters, particularly by the District Ethical Committee. Nurses and other health professionals are not yet seen universally as so reliable, although they remain important secondary gatekeepers.

The need to provide evidence of appropriate levels of support, in order to gain access to records, samples of patients, etc., is one which is frequently overlooked. For an 'outsider', this may cause difficulty in planning the detail of the project and lead to delay or discontinuation. For the health professional, the structures within which one works must be used, sometimes rather tortuously, to gain legitimate access.

Bulmer (1979) discusses the use of computer data in ways not originally intended. Parents signing consent forms for immunization are unlikely to anticipate that their names and addresses will be entered on to the Child Health Computer and used by researchers. Similarly, FHSA databases have been used to identify samples for GP consumer satisfaction surveys (Chapter 4).

Obtaining the sample

Phase One
In Phase One, a sample of 80 children aged 6–12 months (stratified between priority and non-priority areas) was drawn at random from the Child Health Computer database. All health visitors (second-stage gatekeepers) were sent a listing of the sample, with a request to mark any child's name if they felt that a visit would be inappropriate. Seven children were eliminated in this way. The reasons given included the child being on the Child Protection Register or having a severe disability, considerable family involvement with other professionals and a recent family bereavement. Decisions were left to health visitors for two reasons: primarily to avoid unnecessarily restrictive criteria by relying on the judgement of health visitors in individual cases and secondly to maximize

cooperation from colleagues by giving them some involvement in the project. Some 'interesting' cases may have been excluded as a result.

Letters were sent out sequentially, explaining the study and offering an appointment. The aim was to continue sampling until approximately 40 parents, half from priority and half from non-priority areas, had been interviewed. Interviews were completed with 44 parents, all mothers (72% of the 61 approached), of which 41 were usable. Five people had moved away and could not be traced, nine failed to reply to three requests for an appointment and three refused on the doorstep. The participation rates were similar in priority and non-priority areas.

Finch (1984) described the vulnerability and loneliness of women she interviewed and suggested that being a woman interviewing women was important in the response to her study. In this study, I was not only a woman seeking to interview women but also, for some of the time, overtly pregnant, thus sharing at least in part their status as a parent. This may have contributed to the relatively high participation rate.

Phase Two
In Phase Two, the process of recruitment and access was different and raised other issues. The sample of mothers was taken sequentially from primiparous women attending one consultant's weekly clinic session. Sampling from other sites would have improved the generalizability of the findings, but was ruled out as too time-consuming.

The actual process of access to clients was complex. I attended all ante-natal clinics held by the consultant concerned over a four-month period. Each primiparous woman attending for an appointment between 28 and 32 weeks' gestation and living in Newcastle was identified. I attached a request for inclusion to the notes. Whichever doctor saw her, usually not the consultant, would decide whether or not she should be included (acting as a secondary gatekeeper). Two women were excluded in this way, because of severe problems with the pregnancy.

The attending midwife would then send the woman through to see me, in a small office hung with white coats and stethoscopes. The recruitment rate among women approached in Phase Two was 83%, and 19 women were interviewed, 10 from non-priority and nine from priority areas. It was intended to interview a health visitor involved with each woman. However, due to practical problems, only 10 health visitors were recruited into Phase Two, five associated with women in priority and five in non-priority areas.

Phase Two had a longitudinal design. Clients and health visitors were interviewed three times over the 10 months of data collection, once ante-natally when 28–32 weeks pregnant, then about two and seven months postpartum. Three women and two health visitors subsequently dropped out of the study. The women had all experienced changed circumstances, e.g. moving home, and failed to respond to efforts to maintain contact.

One health visitor dropped out due to illness and one due to the withdrawal of her client.

Methods

Phase One

Interviews

Phase One interviews were carried out in mothers' homes, were tape-recorded and lasted about an hour (range, 30–90 minutes). A semi-structured format was used, with the flexibility to add additional questions. Topics covered included ideas about health, perceptions of the health of their own child, experiences of child health services and perceptions of their health visitor, including feelings about their most recent contacts, general views, how far they felt that the health visitor fulfilled the role they had expected and what changes they would like to see in health visitors' activities.

Photographs of a health visitor talking to a family were used to encourage mothers to discuss their perceptions of health visiting in general. Towards the end of the interview, a list of topics based on Orr's (1980) study was used to see if subjects which had not been mentioned up to that point had ever been discussed with the health visitor.

After six interviews had been completed, additional questions were added, examining health advice and advisers in more depth, an important emergent theme.

Diaries

The diary consisted of three sides of A4 paper, on which parents were asked two questions. Question one asked 'How has the baby been this week?' Question two asked them to complete one section for each time they were in contact with health services during the week. Each section asked them to identify the service, say why they were in contact, describe what happened and indicate how they felt about it.

Phase Two

Interviews with parents

The first interviews with parents in Phase Two, conducted at home during the antenatal period, lasted about 30 minutes and focused on their expectations about their first child. Areas covered included perceptions of significant factors influencing the baby's health, how the mother would decide if the baby was in good health and likely sources of help and advice. Subsequent interviews were modelled on those used in Phase One. The second parent interview, around five months later, built upon the first in various ways, for instance by exploring aspects of health services mentioned in the earlier interview.

After two interviews had been completed at this stage, an additional question was added to the second schedule asking mothers how they had found the process of having the baby. This proved to be a more natural lead in to the next question, about parenting. Most women responded with quite an extensive answer, relaxing and appearing to accept subsequent questions well.

The third interviews took place another five months on, by which time I was conscious of viewing health visiting from a rather more client-centred perspective, having analysed the earlier interview material. This may to some extent have affected the way I approached the later interviews. For example, awareness of the issue of legitimation in earlier client responses made it possible to pick up and explore this idea when it arose in Phase Two.

Interviews with health visitors

Health visitor interviews were conducted about two weeks after the parent had been interviewed at each stage of Phase Two. The interview schedule was based upon that used for parents, modified for professionals in discussion with colleagues from social work and medicine. Topics covered included the health visitor's concept of the role, contact patterns, priorities for visiting, areas of work which she would like to develop and her account of her most recent contact, if any, with the client. Health visitors were asked, like clients, to describe what might be happening in photographs of a health visitor talking to a family and to discuss actual and possible communication with the client about the list of topics derived from Orr (1980).

Longitudinal qualitative research

Little has been written in the methodological literature about repeated interviewing or the effect of longitudinal studies on interviewer–respondent relationships. Laslett and Rapoport (1975) suggest that repeated interviewing enables the researcher to generate a collaborative approach to the research, in order to gain more information, in greater depth than might be the case in a more traditional hierarchical relationship between interviewer and respondent. They advocate interviewers responding to interviewee reactions to the interview situation, rather than trying to eliminate them as undesirable. Oakley (1981b) points out the difficulty in maintaining a detached relationship when there is more than one interview. This was borne out by my experience in the two phases of this study. In the later stages of Phase Two, respondents appeared more relaxed and tended to talk more freely and at greater length than in the earlier stages or Phase One.

The identity and diplomatic problems associated with the researcher 'going native' in response to exposure to user perspectives are mentioned in Chapters 2, 4 and 8. There are particular problems when the researcher belongs to the professional group which is being researched. As a professional, I was still on the margins of understanding clients' views, however much empathy I felt I had developed over a series of interviews and even though I too was a parent sharing some of their experiences.

My exposure to client perspectives led me to see the familiar in a new and critical way. This does not sound too problematic. One should always be willing to grow and develop professionally. But the structure may not be ready to change, or one might be more aware of one's colleagues' and one's own shortcomings, yet relatively powerless to deal with them.

For health professionals working in a bureaucracy, perhaps doing research at fieldworker level, this process can be painful. As Hughes (1960) points out: 'A person cannot make a career out of the reporting of reminiscences unless he is so far alienated from his own background as to be able to expose and exploit it before some new world with which he now identifies himself' (p. ix–x).

RESULTS

Introduction

Analysis of the interview transcripts and diary material followed the 'grounded theory' approach (Glaser and Strauss, 1967; Strauss, 1987). Glaser and Strauss saw the process of theory generation as a progression from raw data to categories (concepts), their properties and then to substantive grounded theories. As concepts emerge, Glaser and Strauss suggest, they indicate areas for further data collection, the process of 'theoretical sampling'. Comparison of essentially similar groups (such as parents of children in the same age group) will lead to a relatively simple theory, whereas comparison of different kinds of group will lead to more wide-ranging theories.

In the present research, the process of analysis and theory generation was not straightforward. It resembled the process of doing a jigsaw without a picture of the completed puzzle, with the solver needing to discover the overall shape while at the same time locating individual pieces correctly. Similarly, the researcher who is attempting to discover a grounded theory must look for an overall pattern of links between concepts and at the same time attempt to locate the detail. As theoretical understanding develops, further examination of the data shades in the gaps in the categories and their properties and helps to establish or strengthen links, making the substantive theory stronger overall.

The analysis below presents a representative picture of themes, perspectives and development. Differences between individuals and the small differences which were found between priority and non-priority areas (Pearson, 1988) are not discussed in this chapter, due to space limitations.

Eight main concept areas emerged from the interview data in this study. They were:

- health, health problems and other concerns;
- the need for help and locating the problem;
- knowledge and experience;
- legitimation;
- advice, support and comparing notes;
- choosing a helper;
- relationship- or problem-centred;
- power and control.

Some of these themes were externally determined by the interview structure. The interview contained questions likely to generate answers in specific terms. For example, material coded as 'health, health problems and other concerns' was usually raised in response to a question about the child's health. However, some themes relating to these concept areas also arose spontaneously in response to other questions, so that they were only partially externally determined.

Other concepts, for example 'legitimation', arose internally from the respondents themselves. These concepts may be seen as having a greater validity than those which are solely externally generated when the purpose is to consider the client's perceptions. Legitimation took different forms at different stages of parenthood. For example, some women expecting their first baby were reassured by their mothers that anxiety about their competence was normal and that they would gain confidence through experience. A mother with an older baby was told by the doctor that her anxiety about the baby vomiting was normal and so legitimate even though there was no health problem. Health professional tolerance of parental anxiety is also discussed in Chapter 3, in the context of accident and emergency departments.

The development of parents

The substantive theory which was arrived at with the help of six case studies (Pearson, 1991) suggested that the nature of parents' previous knowledge and the nature of the problems they encounter influence their choice of helper and the degree of parental control at each stage. While the relationship between these elements remains broadly similar, the balance between them shifts.

At the earliest stage at which data was collected (28–32 weeks pregnant) the situation for parents expecting their first baby was characterized by uncertainty about possible problems or resources. Even the types of problem to be faced were indistinct. Many first-time parents had little common-sense knowledge about childcare and generally relied on professional knowledge, whether from books, midwife, GP or clinic. They had little notion of the problems they were likely to encounter but visualized themselves as having a measure of control in dealing with them.

I would be inclined to think it out for myself. (C)

Professionals were described in ways which indicated that they might perform a 'pathfinder' role, but little detail was given.

[The health visitor will say] This is what we're looking out for.... [She will have] more time to sit and go through things with you. (A)

First-time parents who had had previous experience (for example caring for their own siblings) had some idea of the types of problem they would meet. They expected to maintain their independence, supported by more experienced lay helpers. Power remained with them.

I don't ask anyone else [than mother] now, so why should I start now, just got to get on with it? (C)

The situation was different at the second stage of data collection (8–10 weeks postpartum). Problems requiring help were seen as important. Sometimes they caused panic.

About two weeks after she was born, I noticed [symptoms], and I had an immediate panic, so I phoned the health visitor. (J)

Common-sense knowledge was restricted, but was being acquired quite rapidly. The definitional boundary between normal and abnormal problems was fuzzy.

We've asked the health visitor things, like when she's been sick after feeds. (F)

Professional help was sought predominantly to resolve the boundary between normal and abnormal, in the above case in relation to levels of vomiting. Professional direction was accepted as a means of defining the problem.

I needed someone to tell me. (J)

Even parents with prior experience relied quite extensively on professionals for help and advice, for example about feeding patterns. Each interaction with the professional helped parents to build up or confirm their own knowledge about health and health need, e.g. that a rash wasn't important or that a vomiting episode was.

By the third stage of data collection (7–8 months postpartum), first-time parents could discriminate a much wider range of problems. They had increased both their common-sense and 'professional' knowledge.

Normal and abnormal had become more clearly differentiated. Their skills in coping with problems had developed. Alongside this, their self-confidence as parents had increased.

> With experience, we have realized that they [spots] will go in a few days. (K)

> I think as the baby gets a bit older, you just get more confident, you know, that you can rely on yourself. You can handle problems. (H)

Parents now looked for more reciprocal relationships than those they felt they could establish with health visitors.

> With friends you sort of compare notes. (I)

Where professional help was sought, the desire to retain some control influenced the choice that was made.

Health visitor perspectives

Health visitors' perceptions of health, of problems, of legitimation and of their own role influenced their behaviour at each stage and must be examined alongside those of parents. The views of health visitors were essentially dissimilar to those of parents at Stage One of the research, before the birth of their first child. Health visitors placed greater emphasis on children's normal function and development than parents-to-be and less on being happy or 'not crying'.

The views of parents and health visitors were much closer at Stage Two of the research (two months postpartum), though still retaining some dissimilarities. Health visitors and parents focused on practical advice and help the health visitor could give.

At Stage Three of the research (seven months postpartum) dissimilarities in parental and health visitor perspectives were again apparent. There was divergence in issues identified as important. For example, health visitors stressed reaching normative developmental targets, while parents emphasized social and emotional aspects of health. And there was divergence in views about the health visitor's role, with health visitors seeing themselves as judging and checking while parents wanted the health visitor to have a more supportive role. The gap that could occur is illustrated in the following pair of quotes from a mother and her health visitor.

> Both the GP and the health visitor are something completely remote. (D)

> She is very, very open when you get close to her, but it took a while. It took a few visits before she opened up. (D's health visitor)

DISCUSSION

Developmental issues

The development of the individual as a parent encompasses changes in knowledge and experience, altered understanding of health and health problems and a changing need for legitimation. In addition, parents' need for advice, support or comparing notes varies, depending upon their level of confidence in themselves as parents.

The development of the parent is intimately bound up with that of the child. Initial concepts of health and health problems, based on little or no direct knowledge, give way to the reality of a child whose major demands are functional. A functional approach to health and health problems is adopted. As the child grows and develops, becoming by seven to eight months a more social being, the parents' concepts of health also alter, to become focused more strongly on social/emotional ideas of health. As the child grows older, larger and visibly stronger, some of the anxieties of the early weeks and months, about cot death or about infection, for example, are diminished, reducing the need for reassurance and increasing parental confidence.

The development of the health visitor–client relationship can be seen alongside the development of the child and the development of the parent. Parents value the development of a relationship with the health visitor. Where one was successfully established, they felt close even when actual contact was limited. Where a relationship did not develop, even apparently parallel perspectives could not produce closeness. The development of a relationship was also linked to the management of power and control. Where the health visitor appeared to match her approach to that of the parent, whether for self-determination or for direction, a good relationship usually developed. It was not clear whether a good relationship enabled parent and health visitor to match their approaches more closely, or *vice versa*.

Clients and health visitors – the future?

Individual parents and health visitors themselves differ. In this chapter, it has only been possible to represent 'typical' views. The study suggests that the perceptions of health visitors are, at many stages, different from those of their existing main group of clients. Understanding how these differences occur can help the practitioner to make appropriate interventions. Knowing what clients value, and when they are most vulnerable helps health visitors to identify where they should be working.

Clients are often seen only as 'wanting' services, and not as having a clear pattern of need, the reasons for which can be identified. Bradshaw (1972) distinguishes felt, expressed, normative and comparative needs. Health visitors do not examine or value the felt and expressed needs of the client as much as normative or comparative needs which can be standardized and measured. An approach focused on client perspectives enables the client herself to construct much of the material from which needs and reasons can be extracted.

However, perhaps most important in the new NHS is a return to the question, 'Who is our client?'. In the first Griffiths (1983) era, when this research was being carried out, the client or consumer was undoubtedly the patient. As we move through the nineties, the proxy clients are now District Health Authority purchasing divisions and GPs, particularly fundholders. These clients will undoubtedly have rather different perceptions of health visiting to parents. Without a clear understanding of what health visiting can offer, however, these clients could decide to purchase an inadequate service. They will not really suffer. Only the patients will.

Health needs are being increasingly 'targeted' by professionals. Searching out health needs and facilitating health enhancing activities are, perhaps, no longer quite enough (Traynor, 1993). Productivity, with health implicitly defined as a product, is now the requirement. Lay people's own agendas, demonstrated by this study as often quite different from that of health professionals, may fall by the wayside.

CHAPTER 7

One foot on the escalator: elderly people in sheltered accommodation

Nigel Davison and Jan Reed

INTRODUCTION

The needs of the elderly

The number of elderly people is increasing in industrialized societies, including the UK, and they are becoming a bigger proportion of the population (Central Statistics Office, 1986). This trend has been viewed with alarm by some health care professionals (Luker, 1982; Health Advisory Service, 1982). The medical profession has expressed particular concern about the increase in numbers of frail elderly individuals in need of constant attention, and of those suffering from senile dementia (Chapter 8), for which there is no cure (Brotherston, 1976). People aged 80 and over use health and social services more than their younger peers (Social Services Committee, 1982; Audit Commission, 1986).

Moreover, people of retirement age figure prominently among the deprived and the disadvantaged in the United Kingdom. They are heavily over-represented in substandard housing and are among those most in need of support from the personal social services (Bond and Coleman, 1990).

A number of factors have combined to shift the emphasis in policy away from institutional care to what is loosely called 'care in the community'. One factor has been the general reaction against institutional care (Tinker, 1984). A consultative document (DHSS, 1981) discussed the potential for transferring elderly people from residential care into the community.

The NHS is now placing increasing emphasis on meeting the needs of 'consumer' groups (Horrocks, 1985; DOH, 1989). Programmes to meet the needs of the elderly, however, seem mainly to involve mechanisms for 'screening', 'assessment' or 'case finding'. Such programmes attempt to identify unmet needs, but are health-professional-dominated in the ways that needs are defined and matched to services.

Poulton (1984) provides an example of this type of programme, in which health professionals interpret clients needs in terms of cause, symptoms, illness and cure, i.e. in terms of the medical model. The aim was to formulate an assessment tool and nursing care plan for the elderly, based on patients' (as opposed to nurses') perceptions of need. Poulton found that health professionals' perceptions of client need were quite different from those of clients. Clients interpreted their state of health or illness in terms of disability and the effects this would have on their lives, while health professionals focused on clinical conditions. Byrne (Chapter 3) reports a similar difference in the perspectives of health professionals and patients in accident and emergency departments.

Information about consumer views on health and social services for the elderly is most conspicuous by its absence. Dingwall (1977) commented, while studying the social organization of health visitor training, that student health visitors did not like visiting the elderly because 'it took too long'. Some professionals, perhaps, viewed the eliciting of information from the elderly as a laborious and unproductive task.

The ageing process is portrayed in our culture through images ranging from the wisdom of experience at one end of the spectrum to uselessness and semi-idiocy at the other. The latter notion is probably the most predominant in current culture, with the old seen as functionally and intellectually incapable. If these are the prevailing images of the elderly, then the 'consumer view' is not likely to be assiduously sought and policies and service provision will be based primarily on organizational and professional views.

These views seem to involve a notion of increasing dependency as the elderly grow older, with services organized correspondingly. Eley and Middleton (1983) describe the continuum of care as beginning with services for 'minor' health problems, generally provided outside hospitals to clients living in their own homes. As health needs and dependency increase, the elderly progress along the continuum, receiving more and more professional intervention and spending less and less time in their own homes. Eventually, they leave their original home and live in specially adapted accommodation. This is, however, not the end of the continuum. As dependency increases, the elderly client can move through other types of accommodation, e.g. residential care homes, ending up in a hospital bed.

The problems with this model are readily apparent. The client is expected to move to services, potentially a stressful process, involving the disruption of social and family networks. Indeed, as Eley and Middleton (1983) point out, an elderly person may move home several times in their last few years, when they are likely to be least resilient. For those who have lived in their own home for many years, such changes must seem bewildering, requiring great personal adaptation.

More fundamentally, perhaps, this model seems to be based on the assumption of a one-way movement through levels of dependence. Elderly clients are implicitly expected to become more and more dependent as time goes on. The model fails to recognize that dependency may decrease or may be episodic, and that people will need services that match complex trajectories. It may also generate a self-fulfilling prophecy, if service provision undermines or prevents potential returns to independence.

In Chapter 2, the idea of an escalator of care is discussed in relation to systems of care designed to deal with dependency. Embarking on a career as a client of services for the elderly can be compared to stepping onto an escalator. There is only one direction to go, towards greater dependence. Getting off is difficult. One's involvement is passive and one is carried along by the system.

Sheltered accommodation

Sheltered accommodation can be seen as one of the first steps on the escalator of care. It gained rapidly in popularity in the 1960s and 1970s, as a form of social provision for elderly people in which clients are housed in purpose-built accommodation with a central warden system. This warden system provides a 'safety net' for residents. If they are ill or need help, there should be someone immediately available. Because accommodation was specifically designed for the elderly (with bathroom and kitchen adaptations, easy access and no stairs), it was hoped that problems, particularly accidents, would be minimized.

Sheltered housing was seen to combine housing with care, to provide support whilst fostering independence and to allow flexibility and experimentation in adapting schemes to local circumstances. By the late 1970s hundreds of schemes were running, occupied by half a million elderly tenants (Bond and Coleman, 1990). Extravagant expectations were aroused and sheltered accommodation was regarded by some as the solution to a range of complex problems.

The move to sheltered accommodation may be made on 'health grounds', if the elderly person has health problems which have resulted in dependence on services to maintain daily activities or if their health problems are such that they are felt to need closer monitoring.

Although medical problems may lead to the move into sheltered housing, this service is primarily one which provides functional and social support rather than medical care. A person with arthritis, for example, will not receive any additional medical treatment by virtue of being in sheltered accommodation. Rather, they will receive more support in coping with the problems caused by arthritis, such as reduced mobility. Decisions about entry into a range of services will depend as much on the person's perceived circumstances – e.g. ability to cope with disability, informal carer support – as on their medical condition. Health, therefore, is not the primary concern of sheltered accommodation, but it underpins the way in which it is allocated and used.

Selection for this type of accommodation is not standardized, and does not usually include a formal assessment of need. Sheltered housing is generally regarded as a place for 'at risk' or vulnerable elderly people (Eley and Middleton, 1983). This leads to an expectation of a higher level of care in sheltered housing than would be expected for an old person living at home. On the other hand, sheltered housing requires residents to have a higher degree of independence than do other forms of institutional care, such as residential care homes.

Little account is taken of clients' needs or capabilities in determining their suitability for sheltered accommodation. Because the services available are based on professional assumptions about the needs of client 'types', those individuals who do not fit neatly into any client category cause problems. The emphasis can be on fitting the client to the service, rather than the service to the client.

METHODOLOGY

Introduction

The aims of the research

The research study, for which fieldwork was carried out in 1988–9, was designed to investigate the experiences and views of clients of services for the elderly, focusing on those who had entered sheltered housing, the point on the service continuum at which the client is required to leave his/her original home. This is a significant step, involving a certain amount of 'burning bridges'. The original home is relinquished, making a return to non-institutionalized care extremely difficult.

The aims of the research were:

- to investigate the perceptions of their health of elderly residents living in sheltered accommodation (residents);
- to explore residents' perceived needs;
- to compare residents' perceptions of their own health with those of wardens.

The sample

Access and gatekeeping

An outline of the intended research was sent to the housing manager of the company who owned the sheltered accommodation selected for the research. She had no objections to the tenants being interviewed, but suggested it would be advisable to contact the warden first who 'may be able to suggest tenants who would be most cooperative'.

This suggested a possible gatekeeping problem since 'uncooperative' tenants might have been those who were most unhappy about their situation. With the assistance of the head warden, a complete list of current residents was compiled. During the compilation of this list, the warden began to identify some clients as 'deaf', 'blind' or 'rarely in'. She stated that she could identify at least four clients who, in her view, would not wish to participate in the project. It was possible that the warden's perceptions were based on stereotyping or lack of knowledge, or that she might select residents who would give the most favourable impression of staff–resident relationships. With the warden's agreement, therefore, residents were approached directly.

Approval for the study was obtained from the Newcastle Health Authorities/University of Newcastle Joint Ethics Committee. Although it became apparent during interviews that many respondents had chronic illnesses, for example, rheumatoid arthritis, they were classified as 'healthy volunteers' for the application to the Joint Ethics Committee.

Medical representatives on the committee viewed the respondents as 'potential patients' and were concerned that the researchers would seek access to individuals' medical records. The proposal to the Ethics Committee had to be revised to state explicitly that the intention of the research was not to examine care provided or to describe the characteristics of recipients of a particular service. This problem highlighted Webb's (1984) observation that medical hegemony in the health services results in doctors 'owning' 'their' patients, or even 'potential patients'. Pearson (Chapter 6) encountered similar problems in her research into health visiting.

Ethical issues

Ethical committee guidelines require protection of the health and well-being of human subjects, confidentiality and informed written consent. However, there are other ethical issues not addressed in the rules and procedures of research committees.

The principal researcher (ND) approached possible participants individually and explained the aims of the research. Respondents were given the opportunity to refuse to participate at any stage. An explanation was given as to how the data would be reported and respondents were assured that their names would not be used in the final report. However, there is always a possibility that participants' identities may be inadvertently revealed in the reporting of qualitative data.

As a nurse involved in health and social research, the principal researcher experienced some role conflicts. The researcher was asking the respondents for a great deal of personal information and giving nothing in return, apart from the opportunity for them to express their views. It would have been unfair to simply collect data and make no response to any questions asked by the respondents. However, it would have been unethical for the researcher to collude with criticisms of service provision made during the interviews.

Obtaining the sample

A convenience sample was taken for this exploratory study. This sampling technique did not seek to represent the population of elderly people in sheltered accommodation. Therefore, the generalizability of the results is limited. The group chosen for interview was all the elderly people residing in one sheltered accommodation scheme in the west end of Newcastle-upon-Tyne. As only one setting was sampled, the research should be treated as a case study. The results cannot be generalized to other sheltered accommodation schemes.

Of 27 residents, 21 (70%) agreed to participate in the research. Of these 21, 16 were female and five male. All were aged over 65. The six residents who refused to participate were three married couples, while those who agreed to participate were all living on their own. Those who refused to participate indicated that at the time of the project they felt healthy and did not therefore wish to discuss their health.

Respondents were interviewed individually, within their own flats or bed-sitting rooms, in order to maintain confidentiality. The methodology chosen for the project, single, in-depth interviews, provided a limited time sample, with respondents interviewed on the same afternoon, over consecutive weeks.

Methods

Interviews with residents

The research was exploratory and qualitative, with data collected through in-depth interviews, which were taped and transcribed for analysis. The aim was to explore residents' own perceptions of their health status and needs. Non-directive interviews allowed respondents to take the subject of discussion in whatever direction they preferred. Some responses were constrained by interviewees' physical and mental impairment.

All those interviewed were living on their own and had few opportunities to express their views or ask questions. Some talked at length about a variety of topics. The researcher was able to elicit more specific information from respondents by careful probing. The average interview time was about one hour (range 25–90 minutes).

Interviews took the form of informal discussions. Respondents were encouraged to talk about things that most concerned them, but the interviewer's opening remarks remained constant: 'Could you tell me where you were living before you came to this accommodation and the reasons which led you to apply?'. Ideas which clients raised during an interview could be tested out in later interviews, if the opportunity presented itself. For example, one respondent developed the theme of need and current health status in terms of the implications for her future needs and care. This was an area which had not been considered at the outset of the interviews, but one which was obviously important to the respondent.

This progression from one interview to the next fitted the model of grounded theory (Glaser and Strauss, 1967). Progression was not consistent throughout the interviews. Some categories (perceived needs and health status) had been identified in advance. Although the researcher tried to avoid having preconceptions about the research area, we always know something already and this knowledge affects what we come to know next (Kaplan, 1964).

Interviews with wardens

The head and relief wardens were interviewed about their general perceptions of residents' health status and needs, and their own roles. Interviews were again conducted individually and privately and were taped and transcribed. The main aim was to compare their views on these issues with those of residents. The wardens were interviewed before the residents.

RESULTS

Introduction

Interview transcripts were analysed in order to identify themes and concepts (Strauss and Corbin, 1990). Although the interviews had not explicitly used a biographical or life history approach, the data revealed that the respondents had given historical accounts of their experiences of sheltered accommodation. As the use of chronological referents is an 'everyday' way of describing events, it is not surprising that the interviewees organized their responses in this way.

However, many respondents had at least two histories to tell, the history of their entry to sheltered accommodation, and the history of their health problems. These histories were related, but did not always correspond exactly. The interview data were placed into three categories.

- **routes of entry** – the respondent's and warden's descriptions of the respondent's mode of entry into sheltered accommodation;

- **reasons for acceptance** – the reasons respondents gave for accepting accommodation, even if they had not formally applied for residence;
- **levels of disability and functional status** – respondents' health status and its affects on activities of daily living, as seen by respondents and wardens.

Route of entry into sheltered accommodation

When residents were asked how they applied for sheltered accommodation, their descriptions of the process often differed from those of the warden. Although some residents had been responsible for formal applications, many had not themselves applied. Their route of entry was often unclear.

> I don't know whether it was the doctor or what. Some authority stepped in.

The warden, however, identified two modes of application, formal application by the resident or referral from a social worker.

> Right, there is two or three ways that they can go round [apply]. The main one is ringing the council, or [company providing sheltered accommodation], or any housing people. A form is sent out, they fill in the form, it's sent back to the housing association, and then a local representative goes out and interviews them. The other way [entry route] is through social workers.

This account suggests that the warden saw the client as the 'main' instigator of a move into sheltered housing. Formal applications, however, were often made by a second party rather than the client. In these cases, sheltered accommodation would be suggested to the respondent and then a formal application would be made on their behalf.

> Me husband had been dead for about 18 months when me oldest daughter thought I should have a move out [of her current home].

> The doctor told us to put me name on one of the sheltered houses [waiting list].

Although some were unclear about how they had been placed in sheltered accommodation, all but one resident indicated that they were happy to move and felt little regret at leaving their homes.

> I was quite happy to come in. It was all done within a matter of a week. No trouble at all.

Although most respondents were happy with the outcome, some did not actively choose sheltered accommodation and did not know about this provision until it was mentioned to them by a relative or professional.

They may have been unaware of, or have not considered, other options open to them. The picture painted is one of elderly people 'going along with' the decisions of others, rather than actively making choices.

Reasons for acceptance

The main reason residents gave for accepting a place in sheltered accommodation was wanting to feel safe from crime and fear of crime. They also wanted the security arising from the knowledge that someone was available, day or night, to hear calls for help. Residents were not necessarily concerned about current, specific health problems. Rather, they adopted a preventative 'just in case' strategy.

> I have that feeling of safety, and you know if anything goes wrong, well you can press a button, and someone comes.

Feelings of insecurity and fear of crime were associated with a sense of isolation. All the respondents had lost a partner prior to being, or while, in sheltered accommodation:

> If I'd been alone [respondent's husband was dead] I would have been terrified to be by myself.

Goldsmith and Thomas (1974) see fear of crime as the cause of self-imposed 'house arrest' among older people. One respondent, when asked what she felt was her biggest problem in living alone, stated:

> Security. I did not have attempted break-ins, but I always felt it could happen. I just had that fear.

A respondent who had lived in an upstairs flat expressed fear of being burgled.

> I used to think, if they got in [burglars], what would I do, I am helpless? I think, once they know you are helpless, they would try and break in.

However, despite this fear, she felt much safer living on the ground floor in sheltered accommodation.

> For all I am downstairs here, I don't worry. I have them locks on the window as well.

There is evidence (Banks, Maloney and Willcock, 1975; Mawby, 1982) that the elderly experience less crime than other age groups. Fear of crime must be distinguished from the risk of crime as a reason for elderly people seeking or accepting entry into sheltered accommodation. However, the impact of actual crime on the elderly should not be underestimated (e.g. reduced resilience to stress and physical injury).

Other reasons for acceptance included unsafe housing, possession of home by landlord for future sale and house and gardens becoming too large to manage. These reasons point to a perceived and actual financial insecurity in elderly people who do not have the financial knowledge or resources to control their future.

The reasons for entry into sheltered accommodation given by the respondents in this study are characterized by a recognition not of the positive benefits of this provision but of the perceived negative aspects of staying where they were. The 'community' in which they lived is portrayed as a dangerous place in which they are vulnerable, and in which they will be given few concessions because of their age. This world may not yet have hurt them, but there is always the possibility that it will at some time in the future, particularly if they become more frail. With such views of their community, sheltered accommodation becomes a refuge from society. Many people with learning difficulties also see the community as a dangerous place (Chapter 10).

Levels of disability and functional status

The diseases associated with old age tend to be chronic conditions, for example, coronary heart disease, rheumatoid arthritis. Illness and disabilities, often multiple, are common results of declining function (Brody and Brody, 1974). The physical pain which an illness produces may not be nearly as intolerable as the dependency it causes. One respondent who had rheumatoid arthritis stated:

> I will have to have someone to dress me, and I am not looking forward to that a bit when you have been so independent. The bare necessities of life, you are robbed of them.

Another respondent with severe mobility problems due to the amputation of a leg stated:

> I don't like to put anybody out. It's awful when you want to do things, and you can't, though. I want to clean this place [her room], and I can't.

Some respondents, coping with severe disability, were not actively seeking help because they saw their medical problems as an unavoidable consequence of their age.

> I've got bad legs, I've got [respondent laughs] bad circulation. I'm 82, so, hell, [laughs again] I can't expect to be full of fitness.

Fatalism, or lack of feeling of control over health and illness, may accurately reflect an individual's personal experience of powerlessness to affect the social forces shaping his or her life.

This perception of problems and disability related to the process of ageing was sometimes reinforced by the views of professional health workers.

[The doctor said], 'There is nothing I can do with people of your age. You know some of them [other residents] can't get out,' meaning that I look well.

Respondents who did not seek help were mostly suffering from long-term health conditions such as chronic obstructive airways disease, angina, arthritis, urinary incontinence, but did not perceive their debilitating effects as a sufficient reason to seek further medical advice or help.

The quotations below illustrate the pervasive notion among residents of health problems that were not illness because, implicitly, they assumed that a low level of background health was normal. Ironically, Pearson (Chapter 6) associates a similar notion with the entry into life. Because babies are assumed to be 'naturally' healthy in our culture, mothers identified a class of health problems that were not illnesses, e.g. the baby vomiting. Elderly people construed their health problems as not illness for the opposite reason, because they regarded certain levels of disability as normal.

Well, when I want him [the GP] I don't send for him unless I am really poorly, you know.

Yes, but it is not a sickness [chronic pain in legs], it is just cramps.

I've always had bladder trouble, from when me second baby was born. I just go on and get on and mind me own business.

Adoption of a very short time frame was one way of coping with a potentially downward future trajectory.

I just live day by day, and see what happens.

Ill health is defined in the context of cultural values and social norms, and is thus a relative concept. Symptoms viewed as signs of ill health in one society are not necessarily seen as such in another. As Kennedy (1983) points out: 'Illness, a central concept of medicine, is not a matter of objective scientific fact. Instead it is a term used to describe deviation from a national norm'.

Respondents perceived themselves as healthy, despite physical problems, because they assumed that growing old was inevitably associated with physical disability and discomfort. They understood health functionally, in terms of the ability to achieve their own goals, goals which were themselves heavily influenced by cultural expectations about ageing. This view of health matches the functional WHO (1986) definition rather than the earlier idealistic version (WHO, 1958), as discussed in Chapter 2.

Residents saw themselves as 'healthy for their age', and were thus using age-related health norms. They could therefore give positive descriptions of their health, despite problems which would be viewed as severe from a medical perspective. A possible advantage for residents of adopting this perspective was that it allowed them to establish a distance between self and decaying physical body. This view fits with the traditional 'medical model' of illness as a force attacking passive victims, but was used by residents for their own purposes, to maintain a positive sense of self.

> Well yes, I have not been too bad. (A lady with chronic rheumatoid arthritis)

> Oh fine, no problems at all. (A lady quite disabled due to a crush fracture of her vertebrae)

The wardens' perspectives
In contrast, the head and relief wardens focused on residents' medical complaints. The head warden saw her role as that of a carer, rather than just someone who conducted a daily check on residents. She appeared to enjoy getting involved in physical aspects of care, and discussed the ill health of clients at length.

> Nearly everyone has a heart complaint, some have sugar, quite a few arthritic and one, unfortunately, had a limb removed because of the sugar. In the two years I have been here it's changed dramatically. Two years on, two years older, the health needs is much higher now. The doctors are being called in more.

The head warden, although medically untrained, assumed that she had control over decisions about seeking medical treatment for residents' problems.

> It's your discretion whether they need a doctor or not.

She also took upon herself a much wider responsibility, based on the belief that she supplied residents with their reason for living.

> If I stopped doing what we are doing, their attitude to life would definitely change. I think we would get a situation where they would say, 'Why are we living?'.

The relief warden's perception of the residents health was that they were 'not too well'.

There was an evident contrast between the wardens' and residents' perspectives. The wardens medicalized residents' problems. The head warden assumed that she had control over residents' illness behaviour and that their lives revolved around her. Residents, in contrast, normalized their problems as an inevitable consequence of old age and actively coped with them in their own way, through fatalism, favourable comparisons with others of the same age, a short time frame and distancing themselves from their ill health.

DISCUSSION

There are methodological problems in gaining access to concepts of health, problems which stem as much from the research approach as from respondents' reticence. There is, perhaps, only so much a respondent feels that he or she 'knows', or perceives as being 'relevant', when questioning is constrained by a single unstructured interview.

Respondents themselves should be enabled to set the research agenda concerning what is important for their health and how they might achieve it. Methods that allow individuals to describe the complexities of their lives, with an appreciation of change over time, will allow documentation of health behaviour in context.

Without knowledge of clients' perspectives, formal carers can identify only their most overt needs. The extent to which any worker can explore individuals' health status, and the environmental and personal factors affecting it, will depend upon the degree to which clients are willing to respond and cooperate. Any seeking out of needs must be a participative process, which takes account of clients' personal philosophies and cultural value systems. While the wardens had a generally poor view of residents' health, the residents themselves often perceived their health status to be good, despite chronic illnesses.

Medical and functional models generate quite different perspectives on health. In this project, the medical model failed to reflect respondent views, although respondents used a medical model when they felt it gave a positive picture of their health. The medical picture was one of multiple degenerating pathology, but respondents regarded their health as good. Their perspectives were influenced by expectations about health and activity in old age and of the roles which were open to them.

The kinds of health problems that respondents considered to be illnesses were those of recent onset that interfered with normal activities. Chronic diseases are common in the elderly and often have a slow, insidious onset. The symptoms tend to persist and do not always limit activity. Consequently, they may not provide much impetus towards seeing a doctor.

'Objective' assessment of levels of dependency amongst the elderly cannot take account of the ways in which they see their own needs. Elderly people should not be regarded as a homogeneous group who face similar problems at the same time of life, and who react to them in the same way. Needs are based on the experience of problems, the timing and severity of which is difficult to predict. Each individual will have different environmental support and differing ideas about what is an acceptable quality of life.

One worrying finding of this research is that many residents had not actively sought a move into sheltered housing, but had complied with the decisions of others. Some residents might not have chosen this service if other options had been available and if they had been aware of them. Although residents had few complaints about their situation, their discussions focused on the evils that they had avoided by admission rather than on benefits gained. There needs to be a more careful assessment of clients and an effort to make services more flexible to meet their needs.

Ambiguity in usage of the term 'community' in discussions of 'community care' has often been pointed out (Chapter 1). Like the adults with learning difficulties whose views are considered in Chapter 10, respondents in this study had largely negative views of 'the community' and saw themselves as potential victims of crime and neglect. It is beyond the remit of any health or social services agency to encourage collective social responsibility for the elderly. But measures taken to protect the elderly from crime and to give them financial security might address their problems more directly than the drastic step of placing them in sheltered housing.

This step is drastic because it is very difficult for residents to return to their original home or to another form of independent living if they so wish. The only movement facilitated by service provision is into environments which are increasingly protected and distanced from the rest of the community, e.g. residential or hospital care.

There were systematic differences between resident and warden perspectives on residents' needs. Residents minimized and normalized their medical problems. They saw their needs in terms of maximizing independence while avoiding perceived dangers associated with crime and medical emergencies (as distinct from chronic disability). The wardens' perspectives did not correspond to the idealized version put forward by Heumann and Boldy (1982) who suggest that the concept of warden 'covers all the counselling and organizer roles typically covered by several people assigned to sheltered accommodation.... [It is] designed to produce a close friend and neighbour of the elderly tenants while the tenants are still active and independent; and an advocate and family proxy, in place of a professional health or social service bureaucrat.'

Entry into sheltered accommodation is a decisive move in an elderly person's life up the 'escalator of care', a move which should not be taken lightly, or without full consultation with the person involved. To do otherwise, as appears to have occurred with the people in this study, is to impose professionally and organizationally defined indicators of need on the people whom professionals and organizations are ostensibly supposed to serve.

CHAPTER 8

Care of elderly people suffering from dementia and their co-resident informal carers

Charlotte L. Clarke

INTRODUCTION

This chapter discusses the implementation and results of a study of relationships between the dementing elderly and their informal and formal carers. The study began in 1988 in Newcastle upon Tyne. Data was collected by means of interviews with informal carers, informal carer diaries, questionnaires completed by formal carers and case studies of informal carers with all their formal carer contacts.

The chapter is organized into three main parts. Firstly, dementia and informal caregiving are considered as health care issues. Secondly, the methodology of the study is discussed. Problematic issues for this research are referred to, particularly gatekeeping and non-participation. Thirdly, some results from the study are discussed, organized around the core construct of 'normalizing'.

Prevalence of dementia

Understanding the impact which dementia has on the individual and those they interact with requires more than purely pathological representation. The difficulty in identifying just what dementia is and how severely it affects the individual's life means that an absolute picture of its prevalence cannot be obtained. A diagnosis of dementia depends on an arbitrary dividing line drawn at some point in a continuum of disability. 'Prevalence' will depend upon where that line is drawn. The problem of classifying marginal cases is found for other kinds of chronic conditions which are defined functionally, for example alcoholism (Chapter 9), learning difficulty (Chapter 10) and mental illness (Chapter 11).

Hofman *et al.* (1991) reviewed 23 European epidemiological studies of dementia. They conclude that the prevalence rises from 1.0% in those 60–64 years old to 32.3% in those 90–94 years old, the figures nearly doubling with every five years of increase in age.

Community care

Service provision

People with dementia and their informal carers have varied contact with statutory services and receive different mixtures of health and social service care. Dementia sufferers may be passed from service to service in an attempt to shift both the financial liability and the stresses associated with working with such people (Badger, Evers and Cameron, 1989).

Statutory service provision takes various forms. Examples include screening programmes in primary care that seek to detect undiagnosed disease (MacLeod and Mein, 1987), flexible home care (Murphy and Rapley, 1986) and decentralized community management through key workers (Challis *et al.*, 1987).

The current policy of community care, building on the Griffiths Report (1988b), serves to encourage the maintenance of the dementing person at home. This policy can be contrasted with the high profile of medical and institutional involvement in maternity care (Chapter 5).

Care of the informal carer

The care of dementing people in the community cannot be discussed without considering the role and needs of their informal carers. Co-resident caregivers in Britain, now estimated to number 1.7 million (Redding, 1991), are involved in an increasing amount of health care activity. Statutory services have long been asking themselves just who they are providing a service for, and recent government publications have placed care of the informal carer high on the agenda (DOH, 1989).

There are several forms of service provision that have as their primary objective support of the informal carer. These include day and residential respite schemes (Donaldson *et al.*, 1988) and carer support groups (Haley *et al.*, 1987). However, Twigg (1989) argues that some forms of care are unresponsive to the varied needs of informal carers.

Effects of caregiving on informal carers

There is strong empirical evidence that caring can have a detrimental effect on the carers' health, particularly their emotional health (e.g. Nolan, Grant and Ellis, 1990). However, the level of informal carer stress is not directly related to the severity of disability in the dementing person, because of the mediating effect of other factors (Parker, 1990). Adaptive coping strategies include seeking social support (Neundorfer, 1991) and positive reappraisal of the situation (Nolan, Grant and Ellis, 1990). The carer's interpretation of his/her role in caregiving is more significant than specific problems such as incontinence.

Formal carer support for informal carers

Informal carers try to 'make sense' of their situation, to re-establish predictability and control over their lives. Not knowing what to expect or how to interpret events have been found to be major problems for them (Wilson, 1989).

Counselling can help informal carers to cope with stress (Toseland *et al.*, 1990). Increasing the amount of instruction and information may reduce feelings of helplessness (Williams and Fitton, 1991). However, descriptions of the 'typical' course of dementia risk overlooking the variability of its progression, and of the associated problems (Lynott, 1983).

Bond (1992) argued that the care of people with dementia has been medicalized. For informal carers, medicalization allows a structure to be applied to care and legitimates bizarre behaviour. But medicalization leads to a focus on the dementing person's symptoms and obscures the social context, for example, the influence of the circumstances of care giving and the caregiving relationship. The research discussed in this chapter used informal carers' own frameworks for understanding their relationship with the dementing person. It will be argued that service interventions sometimes disrupt informal carer attempts to normalize relationships.

METHODOLOGY

Introduction

Data was collected in three main phases. In Phase One, 14 informal carers were interviewed in their own homes about their caring role and its impact on their lives. These informal carers kept diaries for one week. In Phase Two, a sample of 60 formal carers completed postal questionnaires about their support for informal carers and dementing people, and about potential conflict between the needs of these two groups. In Phase Three, nine case studies were compiled. Interviews were carried out with the informal carer, who also kept a diary, and with all 25 formal carers involved with the families.

The sample

Defining the population

Criteria for identifying dementing people

The identification of a sample of dementing people is complicated by the uncertain relationship between pathology and cognitive and behavioural problems experienced. Researchers can draw on two approaches to identify samples.

Firstly, psychometric tests may be used (Haley *et al.*, 1987) to assess cognitive disability. The disadvantages are that 'the problem' is located entirely in the dementing person and divorced from its social context, and that correct classification depends upon the reliability and validity of the test.

The second approach, adopted for the present study, is to treat dementia as a social construct. Dementia is not considered in terms of pathophysiology but as a socially defined experience. The disadvantage of this approach is that it will not detect cases of underlying disease that have not been labelled as dementia.

In this study, individuals were classified as dementing if their formal carer and GP thought that they had dementia. There were a few instances in which the GP did not confirm the presence of dementia, considering the person to be depressed, for example. Formal carers and the GP did not always share the diagnosis of dementia with the individual or their informal carer, who sometimes attributed the cognitive and behavioural changes to 'just getting old'.

Criteria for identifying informal carers

There are also problems in determining which members of the dementing person's social network should be classified as informal carers. The clearest division is between those carers who are co-resident, as in this study, or not co-resident. However, other issues might be raised, including the quantity of caring required before someone becomes classified as an informal carer and the kinds of caring required. Caring for someone with a mental impairment often involves supervision and observation rather than 'hands on' physical care.

People looking after a relative may not see themselves as carers and may simply interpret their actions as part of their marital or filial relationship. By defining themselves in this way, informal carers may be attempting to normalize relationships with the dementing person. Bell, Gibbons and Pinchen (1987) suggest that carers are inclined to centre activity on the confused person rather than themselves.

Locating the sample

Locating and obtaining access to a sample are usually difficult in community settings. A number of studies describe outreach methods, for example 'advertising' through local newspapers, radio stations, support groups and community centres (Chenoweth and Spencer, 1986). While sampling from established groups does provide easy access to a large number of caregivers, they are likely to be caregivers who are established in that role, who are aware of their own needs and who have the initiative to join such groups. Outreach methods appear to be less successful in Britain than the USA (Bell, Gibbons and Pinchen, 1987), possibly due to varying perceptions of a 'carer', lack of assertiveness in self-referral and the perceived 'private' nature of caregiving in British culture.

In Britain, samples appear to be more efficiently selected through specific services, for example day hospitals (Gilhooly, 1984) and third party contacts, particularly professionals (Clarke and Watson, 1991). However, this procedure again reaches only a proportion of informal carers: those who are in receipt of services. Carers who have, perhaps through choice, 'slipped through the net' or who are caring for a dependant who is too mildly or too severely impaired to utilize the service are unlikely to be identified.

Pilot work for the present study, in one electoral ward of Newcastle upon Tyne, demonstrated that each statutory or voluntary service knew of a relatively discrete group of dementing people. There appeared to be little multidisciplinary knowledge of any one individual. The sample was therefore drawn from multiple sources, including health visitors, district nurses, community psychiatric nurses, social workers, home carers, domiciliary workers employed by voluntary organizations, staff in day centres (health and social services), residential homes and hospital wards.

Two criteria were used in sample selection. Firstly, the referring service had to consider that the individual had dementia. Secondly, the dementing person had to have a co-resident informal carer. Conformity to these two selection criteria was established by a check with the dementing person's GP.

Negotiating with gatekeepers

Contacting informal carers via services required the agreement of 'gatekeepers' who Burgess (1984) described as 'those individuals in an organization that have the power to grant or withhold access to people or situations for the purposes of research' (p. 48). The quality of the access negotiated has a direct effect upon the quality of the eventual research project, particularly in primary care settings (Murphy, Spiegal and Kinmonth, 1992). This stage of the research involves a certain amount of 'selling yourself'. It is important to appear confident and familiar with the proposed work (Taylor and Bogdan, 1984).

There are three key issues to be considered in relation to gatekeepers. Firstly, identification of an effective gatekeeper can be problematic, particularly when the researcher is unfamiliar with the management structure, often the case in multidisciplinary research. Some organizations, such as voluntary groups and primary health care teams, have little management hierarchy and may choose to raise the issue of access at their next management meeting, slowing down the research. If the 'wrong' gate-keepers are identified in such organizations, the research may be thwarted after it is well under way (see Chapter 11 for an example).

The second key issue is the need to keep gatekeepers appraised of the progress of the study. Managers may not appreciate the relatively long time-scales of academic research. Unless kept informed, they may come to believe that the project has stalled, or that they are not going to be given any feedback, with implications for their subsequent cooperation.

The third issue is the perception of the researcher's position by others in the organization. The researcher may be seen as allied to gatekeepers in management positions, with damaging effects on the flow of information from those elsewhere in the organizational hierarchy. The researcher needs to gain the trust of fieldworkers and to offer and maintain confidentiality.

The issues which concerned gatekeepers most were the potential quantity of extra work required of staff, and confidentiality, both for clients and the organization. A total of 34 gatekeepers and 17 general practices were contacted during the study. In the majority of cases a straightforward approach to the gatekeeper was sufficient to gain access to the organization, and none of those approached refused access. The gatekeepers were kept in contact with the progress of the study, notified when the data collection was completed in their area, thanked for their assistance and supplied with copies of any reports arising from the study.

Obtaining the sample

Phase One: informal carer interviews and diaries

The approach to the informal carer was made initially by letter, introducing the researcher and briefly outlining the purpose of the study. The letter contained a section for return if the informal carer did not wish any further contact. An informal visit was subsequently made, usually without prearrangement, in which the researcher and informal carer and, on occasions, the dementing person, discussed the study. If the carer wished to participate, the use of a diary was explained and a copy was left with him/her.

The informal visits were valuable for two reasons. They served as preinterviews (Paterson and Bramadat, 1992), enabling the researcher and informal carer to become acquainted with each other 'off tape'. Issues raised at this time could then be discussed in more detail in the taped interview. The visits also allowed the informal carer to establish what was required during the interview. Frequently, informal carers made arrangements for the dementing person to be supervised during the interview.

Of 37 informal carers approached in Phase One, 22% (8) were unable to participate, due to discontinuation of home care of the dementing person. Of the remaining 29 informal carers, 14 (48%) agreed to participate, although two opted not to complete the diary. The final Phase One sample consisted of two men and four women who were caring for their spouse, and one man and seven women caring for a parent. Of those who refused to participate, eight men and five women were caring for a spouse or sibling, while one man and one woman were caring for a parent.

Phase Two: formal carer questionnaires
The formal carers in the sample were employed by the health, social or voluntary services and reflected the wide range of services which have contact with dementing people and their informal carers, for example community nursing staff, social workers, voluntary care workers as well as a range of health and social service staff involved in the provision of day and respite care. Gatekeepers within 21 organizations distributed the questionnaire to the sample, who returned it directly to the researcher by post.

Of 137 questionnaires issued to gatekeepers, 44% (60) were returned. Of the participating formal carers, 38% (23) worked for the social services, 52% (31) for health services and 10% (6) for voluntary services. Within the sample, 87% (52) of formal carers were female and 6% (4) had no formal work-related qualifications.

Phase Three: case studies
In Phase Three, nine case studies were conducted. As described for Phase One, 20 informal carers were identified and approached. Of these, six refused to participate and five were unable to (four because the dementing people died at the time of the study). The participating informal carers were two men and four women caring for a spouse and two men and one woman caring for a parent.

All of the 25 formal carer contacts of the nine informal carers and dementing people were also approached. Their identification depended on close collaboration with gatekeepers, and all 25 approached agreed to participate. The number of formal carer contacts per case ranged from one to five. Of these formal carers, 56% worked for health services, 32% for social services and 12% for voluntary services.

Data collection methods

Introduction

A symbolic interactionist perspective using mainly qualitative methods was employed to explore the complexities of informal carer perspectives. It was not ethically viable to undertake observation of informal carers because of the private nature of community caregiving. Data was collected from informal carers through diaries and interviews. Data was collected from formal carers by means of questionnaires for the Phase Two study and interviews for the Phase Three case studies. The questionnaire was more convenient for formal carers than a prearranged interview, while the case study interviews enabled data to be collected about specific caregiving situations.

The phases of data collection

Phase One: informal carer interviews
In Phase One, data was collected through interviews with informal carers in their own homes and diaries completed during the previous week (discussed subsequently). Interview lengths ranged between half an hour and three hours. Although a prompt sheet was available, there was no standard form or sequence to the questions. Interviews were taped, with respondents' permission, and transcribed for qualitative analysis.

The interviews were particularly valuable in seeking to understand how people made sense of the situations they were in and the issues which were important to them. Information giving often took the form of narration or storytelling (Graham, 1984). Informal carers were encouraged to tell their own story of caregiving. They were allowed to include or omit whatever information they wished and so were afforded some rights of participation. Interviews have a vibrant quality, described by Howarth (1989) as 'rescuing the individual from the crowd and from the stereotype. Suddenly personality, character, warmth and humour sharply replace the amorphous mass' (p. 7).

Phase One: informal carer diaries
Burgess (1984) describes diaries as providing a first-hand account of a situation to which the researcher does not have access and as a complement to data gathered from other sources. The diaries provided valuable concurrent data about the details of caring for a dementing person, and complemented the more retrospective, generalized information obtained from the interviews.

Informal carers kept the diary for seven consecutive days. It had a loosely structured format, inviting comments about the dementing person, themselves, family, friends and any contact with statutory or voluntary services. It was anticipated that the diary would prove unacceptable to some elderly carers and to those who were not confident in their literacy skills. However, only two informal carers declined to complete the diary, citing lack of time as the reason for refusal.

Phase Two: formal carer questionnaires
The questionnaire, completed by 60 formal carers, asked general questions about their attitudes to working with informal carers and dementing

people. Its content was determined by a review of literature, including work on staff burnout (e.g. Astrom *et al.*, 1991) and analysis of the results of Phase One of this study.

The first section of the questionnaire asked about respondents' personal and employment characteristics. The second section had a dual question framework in which 23 statements with a Likert-type response scale were integrated with 36 prompts for qualitative responses (Clarke *et al.*, 1993).

Phase Three: case studies

Nine case studies were compiled from interviews with formal and informal carers and informal carer diaries. Case studies were valuable at this stage of the study because they facilitated the development of the emerging theory (Strauss, 1987). Informal carers were interviewed and completed diaries, as in Phase One, and their formal carers were interviewed.

The interviews with formal carers were conducted in their own workplace or home. The taped interviews were semi-structured and used a laddering process to probe the rationale for particular actions (Pollock, 1986). The interviewees were aware that they would be asked 'why?' on occasions and, perhaps consequently, many volunteered this depth of information without explicit prompting. The interviews lasted between 20 minutes and two and a half hours. They contained three sections: biographical information, general questions about working with dementing people and informal carers and questions specific to caregiving for the case study dementing person and informal carer.

Data analysis

Each phase of the study was analysed before the next was carried out, influencing subsequent data collection. Phase One interviews and diaries were analysed thematically (Clarke, 1989). Phase Two questionnaires were postcoded, and analysed with descriptive statistics. Phase Three case studies were analysed within a grounded theory framework, using open and axial coding to develop theory (Strauss, 1987).

Diagrams and theoretical memos were used to integrate the data from the diaries, interviews and questionnaires and to identify the core category. In this study the core category (Fagerhaugh, 1986) that emerged was the process of 'normalizing' disability.

RESULTS

Introduction

The concept of normalizing has its origins in work on the management of chronic illness (Strauss *et al.*, 1984; Robinson, 1993). It can be described as the way in which the ill person is defined, and continually redefined, as 'normal' by themselves and their family. Identification as being normal enables the dementing person and informal carer to live in a relatively problem-free manner.

Informal carers, sometimes with intervention from formal carers, maintained this process of normalization by employing three strategies: pacing, confiding and rationalizing. However, there were conflicts between the varying perceptions of informal and formal carers. Informal carers tended to aim for problem freedom, to have a present time frame and to be oriented to the person rather than the illness. Formal carers tended towards problem saturation, a future time frame and illness rather than person orientation.

Informal carer normalization strategies

Pacing

One way in which the informal carers sought to manage the demands placed upon them and to maintain a sense of normality was to pace their exposure to them. For example, one informal carer said that he was trying to 'hang on as long as you can'. (Husband S, Phase One interview) Formal carers often attempted to facilitate pacing.

> The primary aim is to relieve the carer and to keep the carer functioning to look after the patient as long as possible. (Community Care Manager, Phase Three interview)

Pacing most visibly involved the utilization of services such as day and respite care.

> A lot of people say to me you should have him put away for good. I says, well, the hospitals are good. They take him for a month, and they give me him back for a month. (Wife P, Phase Three interview)

However, a dilemma for informal carers was that pacing through the use of respite services partially institutionalized the dementing person and so reduced the normality of their relationship. It was sometimes difficult for informal carers to utilize day care and respite services if they had no desire to remove the dementing person from their day-to-day life.

> I feel, why should I have the time off to be enjoying myself, and she's in an institution? (Husband S, Phase One interview)

Pacing also involved the management of emotional involvement with the dementing person.

> I have to laugh or I would cry, and that would not do. But it is sad, and I think, somewhere, in that body, is my husband. (Wife C, Phase One diary)

Confiding

Confiding is a strategy which enables informal carers to identify their problems and look for solutions. It can also help informal carers to maintain a perspective on their lives. In redefining their lives as normal, informal carers seek confirmation that problems are not insurmountable and that their lives are not too dissimilar to others'.

> You get a tremendous lot of help, just by chatting about the problems we have, and how to deal with them. (Wife B, Phase One interview)

Formal carers also believed that enabling informal carers to talk was effective in relieving stress, and helping them to look after the dementing person. There was 'great need for sharing and self-expression' (Psychiatric Day Unit Sister A, Phase Two questionnaire). Formal carers saw informal carers as needing to talk about coping and feelings of loss and futility.

> Problem solving, coping strategies, finding humour in impossible situations, dealing with feelings of living bereavement. (Senior Day Centre Officer, Phase Two questionnaire)

Informal carers frequently identified their confidant as a member of the family, a friend or some other figure rather than a formal carer. The ability to communicate and feel the support of the confidant was more important than their physical presence.

> All our friends have been in today. They all want to help, and, believe me, we need them very much. (Wife C, Phase One diary).

Rationalizing

Rationalizing the situation was another normalizing strategy employed by informal carers. They made sense of their situation in various ways, for example, by relating their present relationship to past experiences.

> For all he goes on the way he does with us, I wouldn't part with him. No, I mean, really speaking, we've went together from being young. Why we keep him is, he was a very good husband to us. (Wife P, Phase Three interview).

One carer made sense of her situation through a negative sense of obligation.

> Sometimes I just want to crawl into bed and stay there, as this situation is so frustrating and depressing. But you can't, as carers are trapped by necessity, and, in a way, emotional blackmail. (Daughter A, Phase One diary)

Helping informal carers to make sense of the situation and of the dementing person's behaviour was one way in which formal carers attempted to support them.

> Generally, I feel that, if people do understand, they are able to cope, it gives them more understanding of the situation than if they don't understand. That's, sort of, a thing I would normally work to, rather than sort of leading people. (Social Worker, Phase Three interview)

Informal and formal carer approaches to normalization

Informal carers' orientation to normalization was not always supported by formal carers. Differences in approach were evident in three main areas. Firstly, formal carers tended to be problem-orientated, while informal carers tried to maintain normality by minimizing the impact of problems on their lives. Secondly, formal carers were more future-orientated than informal carers, seeking to prepare informal carers for their future caregiving role as the dementing person deteriorated, or to relinquish that role. Thirdly, formal carers were illness-orientated, providing clinical expertise. Informal carers were person-orientated, experts in caring for an individual because of their past lives together.

Seeking problem freedom versus *problem domination*

It was a fundamental wish of the co-resident caregivers in this study that the dementing person should be cared for at home. Reasons included a sense of repayment in the relationship, or because home care appeared to be the best option.

> My whole argument is based on the fear that she'd be going into a home where they treated her like lumps of meat. You read in the papers these stories about how they're treated, if I thought the old lady was in a place like that, I wouldn't be able to live with myself. I couldn't do it. (Son M, Phase Three interview).

There was also the wish to hang on to a relationship that was central, and therefore normal, to their own lives.

> I'll never let them take [husband] off us. They can take him away for a month, and give me a rest, but they'll never take him off us. No, no. (Wife P, Phase Three interview).

A normal life was not relinquished even when the dementing person required care beyond the knowledge and ability of the informal carer. Informal carers redefined life with the dementing person into another normality which embraced the difficulties surrounding someone suffering from dementia, and might also have to include the presence of formal carers.

Formal carers, in contrast, sought to 'assess' and, in doing so, looked for the abnormal in the individual. Thus, their perspectives were problem-orientated, dominated by what was wrong in the lives of the dementing person and their informal carers, rather than what was ordinary and normal.

> What we do is, they have a full physical examination, they have their bloods taken, routine dementia screening, they have X-rays, skull, chest, and we have the ECG and EEG done. And basically it's just a case of getting to know them, trying to find out how they interact socially. (Enrolled Nurse, Psychiatric Day Centre, Phase Three interview).

Variations in approach to caregiving were evident in both the initial stages of taking on caregiving and subsequently. It was common for the informal carer to be reluctant to expose the individual as dementing, and to minimize his/her problems. One outcome was a delay in seeking help.

> He didn't want people to know.... He didn't want people to think he was an idiot. (Wife C, Phase One interview).

Future versus *present time orientation*

Formal carers frequently saw their role as one of preparing the informal carer and dementing person for the future (a downward trajectory in the dementing person's condition). Informal carers were more orientated to present events. They did not want to think about changes which would make caregiving at home impossible.

> All the time, along the line, we kept saying, we tried to tell him the next possible step, and what we could do about that, and he kept saying, 'I don't want to know'. So we said, 'Well, fair enough, but just we'll tell you about it anyway.' (Community Psychiatric Nurse, Phase Three interview).

Despite this resistance, formal carers felt that it was part of their role to make informal carers aware of the likely downward trajectory.

> Carers need to be aware of the future prognosis, and potential difficulties, in order that they can prepare themselves for the future. (Occupational Therapist, Phase Two questionnaire).

Illness versus *person orientation*

Informal carers were often concerned to preserve the personal essence of the individual, despite the outward appearance of a demented person.

Ties of kinship and of relationships that predated the dementia meant that the informal carer had knowledge of the individual before he/she was ill.

> I think others feel he is much more senile than he is. I mean, I live with him all the time, and we converse all the time, and if I can't understand what he says we'll have a laugh because he can't always tell me what he wants. (Wife H, Phase Three interview).

As well as being more problem-orientated, formal carers could not share this intimate knowledge base.

Informal carers felt able to provide a special quality of care, because of their personal knowledge of the dementing person.

> I feed her according to how her bowels are. If I think she's got a lot of water infection I'll give her barley as a vegetable. Things like that just can't be done in the hospital. (Daughter G, Phase Three interview).

Formal carers also felt that it was important to personalize care, but could not draw on knowledge of the individual before that person became dementing.

> One of the reasons [for reminiscing] is that everyone's past is important in terms of who you are now. It's a lot to do with your past in terms of self-respect and self-esteem. For me, as a carer, I get a better impression of who I am working with. I think that can affect how you care, I mean knowing someone's values, knowing how they feel. (Day Centre Officer, Phase Three interview).

DISCUSSION

Limitations of the study

All the informal carers in the sample were co-resident, having specifically opted to commence caregiving or simply drifted into it. The sample may have represented informal carers who were more motivated and positive about caregiving than those who were not co-resident. The sample was further affected by a high proportion of informal carers who either refused (about half those approached) or were unable (about one fifth) to participate in the study. This is not unexpected in a client group which has a high mortality rate and a high rate of movement into residential care.

Working with the dementing elderly and their informal carers

To work effectively with the dementing elderly and their informal carers requires an appreciation of their perspectives, and an awareness of the meanings that dementia and caregiving have for them. Formal carer support was only partly compatible with informal carer attempts to normalize the situation through pacing, confiding and rationalizing. Use of respite care, for example, helped informal carers to pace themselves, but threatened their attempts to maintain a definition of their lives as relatively normal.

Differences were evident in the ways in which informal and formal carers approached normalization. Firstly, the problem-orientated approach of formal carers was at variance with the informal carer and dementing person's search for a relatively problem-free life together. Secondly, formal carers were more future-orientated than informal carers, adopting a remit to prepare the informal carer for future options. Thirdly, formal carers had difficulty in appreciating the 'person' behind the dementia. They had no past knowledge of, or shared experiences with, the dementing person. Informal carers, however, tried to retain a sense of the dementing person as an individual.

If the statutory and voluntary services are to work in partnership with informal carers, they need to appreciate the meanings underpinning the caregiving activities of informal carers. The co-resident carers of the dementing elderly in this study wanted to minimize the effects of the dementia on the relationship between the couple. The results support the contention of Strauss and Corbin (1988) about users of community health services, discussed in Chapter 1, that 'their world is not the professional's world and *vice versa*' (p. 42).

CHAPTER 9

The meaning and influence of disulfiram therapy from a client perspective

Tony Machin and Mike Kingham

INTRODUCTION

You can go to the doctor's, and you've got the shakes, or you've got the DTs something horrible. He doesn't really understand what you're going through.... All he knows is that you're drinking too much, and that you should stop it.

(MACHIN, 1993, P. 3)

The above quotation illustrates the gap that clients often perceive between their own perspectives on a drinking problem and those of helpers. Timms and Mayer (1970) argue that unless health professionals have an insight into client views of reality, therapy and intervention are likely to fail. For the person quoted above, drinking is a 'wicked problem'. He has to balance the financial, social and health costs of drinking against the psychological costs of abstinence.

The present chapter will explore this apparent 'gap' in relation to a specific treatment in a particular sphere of therapeutic interventions, that of disulfiram therapy in problem drinking.

Maynard (1992) estimated that the annual 'social cost' of alcohol misuse in the United Kingdom (including costs to industry, NHS costs, material damage, costs related to criminal activities, unemployment and premature death) was over £2 billion.

A variety of agencies, statutory and voluntary, have evolved in response to alcohol problems. Some attempt to influence policy (e.g. Alcohol Concern), and others to directly help individuals with problems (e.g. NHS clinicians, voluntary counsellors). The network of services is not well coordinated. It is based on different definitions of problem drinking and philosophies of treatment. For example, disease/illness-orientated agencies work alongside those who see problem drinking as learned behaviour.

The chapter begins with an outline of disulfiram therapy from a pharmacological perspective and then briefly considers different professional definitions of alcohol problems. Previous research into disulfiram therapy is then briefly discussed. It will be shown that previous research has ignored the disulfiram user's own understanding of what the treatment means. A qualitative research study which examined user perspectives on this drug is then described and a grounded theory model of 'commitment to abstinence' is presented. Finally, the implications of the findings of the study are discussed.

BACKGROUND

What is disulfiram?

Disulfiram (Antabuse) was first reported in clinical use by Hald and Jacobsen (1948). Disulfiram is the generic drug name whilst Antabuse is the most common brand name.

The drug, usually taken orally, produces an unpleasant and potentially dangerous reaction if alcohol is subsequently ingested. The reaction, which is fairly rapid, includes facial flushing, rapid heartbeat, falling blood pressure, nausea and vomiting. The potential for this kind of reaction remains for seven days after disulfiram has been regularly taken.

The rationale for the use of disulfiram is that an individual with an alcohol problem knowingly utilizes it in order to maintain his/her resolve to continue abstinence from alcohol. A tolerance test is often offered, allowing the disulfiram user to experience the effects of drinking a small amount of alcohol in a supervised environment, with nursing and medical staff present for monitoring and safety reasons.

What constitutes an alcohol problem?

The dominant philosophy within medicine, represented by the medical model, has taken a view of drinking which is 'out of control' as being similar to a disease process in the body. Within this model, problem drinking behaviour usually leads to a diagnosis of 'alcoholism', the term also used by the self-help organization Alcoholics Anonymous. Members of Alcoholics Anonymous believe that alcoholism is a disease that causes the drinking behaviour of the affected individual.

Heather and Robertson (1985) concluded from their research review that alcohol problems are not effectively explained by disease or illness models that focus on processes inside the drinker's body (medical 'gaze' is discussed more generally in Chapter 14). These authors argue for a concept of problem drinking as a 'socially learned behavioural disorder'.

The disease/illness approach may lead problem drinkers to see themselves as helpless victims of alcoholism and to pass responsibility for treatment to therapeutic agencies.

There is also controversy about the concept of 'relapse' in problem drinking (Donavon and Marlatt, 1988). Some define relapse as a return to pretreatment levels of alcohol consumption. Others suggest that any alcohol ingestion after a commitment to abstinence by the drinker constitutes a relapse. This issue will be discussed below, from a user perspective, in terms of the idea of the flexible use of disulfiram.

The varying positions adopted by professional clinicians, support agencies and self-help groups with respect to the essential nature of alcohol problems and the range of possible treatments put the problem drinker at the centre of a web of conflicting advice, information and opinion.

What has previous research told us about disulfiram?

A number of research studies have taken a quantitative approach to the evaluation of disulfiram treatment. Critchfield and Eddy (1987) concluded from a review of four American studies that disulfiram treatment is unlikely to increase the probability that a middle-aged 'alcoholic' who accepts treatment will abstain for one year; but that it can be expected to lead to an average increase of 30 in the number of dry days per year, probably leading to health improvements.

Brewer (1986) examined the compliance patterns of 84 British patients who had been offered supervised disulfiram. Over a six-month period, 45% (38) took the drug regularly and remained abstinent and 13% (11) refused to start or dropped out of treatment. The other 42% (35) attempted to evade or sabotage treatment in various ways, e.g. by drinking while taking the drug, or inducing vomiting after ingestion. However, Brewer (1986) reported that, in most cases, clinicians were able to 'outmanoeuvre' their patients by increasing dose and/or adjusting supervision arrangements. The concept of 'outmanoeuvring' patients seems somewhat combative, therapeutically.

Research into the use of disulfiram has mainly focused on quantitative measures, and tells us little about the meaning of disulfiram use from a user perspective. One exception is an American case study by Straus (1974), an account of correspondence over the period 1945–72 with a man who had a chronic alcohol problem and who used disulfiram, unsuccessfully, during the period 1950–1.

Little work has been done in exploring the meaning of disulfiram use from the user's viewpoint. The research described in this chapter (Machin, 1993) was designed to address this 'gap'. The aims of the research may be summed up in the following research question: how does disulfiram therapy help problem drinkers achieve abstinence?

The use of disulfiram can be considered from three different perspectives:

- meaning at the level of clinical practice;
- the meanings and experiences of disulfiram users;
- the meanings attributed to clinicians and users by researchers.

Research and clinical practice have both failed to take account of user perspectives, reinforcing an image of the user as a passive object of treatment. Disulfiram users have had a mainly one-way relationship with those who research them, with user behaviour being 'measured' and 'counted'. Measures of treatment efficacy are defined by clinicians and researchers.

In order to obtain disulfiram therapy, an individual needs to make contact with a prescriber who must accept that person for treatment. Clinicians define and subjectively apply criteria for consideration of disulfiram therapy, e.g. social stability, the availability of a third party to supervise compliance, absence of 'impulsive' behaviour. Disulfiram may thus be seen as more of an option for the therapist than for the client. Researching the meaning which disulfiram has for users may begin to redress the balance towards clients.

METHODOLOGY

Sampling issues: who and why?

Sampling processes in qualitative research differ in purpose from those in quantitative studies. While quantitative sampling is usually concerned with randomness and representativeness, qualitative 'theoretical sampling' may purposively seek out interesting or revealing cases, since it is experiences and events that are being sampled.

The sample for the present study was selected from patients using one NHS community agency based within a large urban area of North-East England. This agency was chosen mainly because the principal researcher (TM) had a good relationship with it.

Agency therapists acted as initial 'gatekeepers' in sampling and identified a number of potential participants who were using disulfiram regularly. All agreed to take part in the study. Ultimately, six male participants were selected. Selection was based chiefly on convenience, availability and willingness to participate. It was also felt that these service users could describe experiences which were fairly typical of service users who were positive about disulfiram.

Two members of the sample were married, two divorced and two single. Their ages ranged from 36–57 years. All were manual or skilled manual workers, but only two were actively employed at the time of interview.

There are many problem drinkers who do not have the degree of 'social stability' required to support disulfiram therapy or even access to helping services, e.g. the homeless 'skid row' problem drinker. However, the sampling policy related to the aims of the study because the research question focuses upon positive outcomes (i.e. how disulfiram helps). No women were included in the sample, though there was opportunity to do so. This sample was constructed to explore in some depth the meaning of disulfiram for service users.

Methods

A grounded theory approach (Glaser and Strauss, 1967) to data collection and analysis was adopted. Strauss and Corbin (1990) describe the essence of this approach as follows: 'One does not begin with a theory, then prove it. Rather one begins with an area of study and what is relevant to that area is allowed to emerge' (p. 23). The initial area of study was user perspectives on the drug disulfiram. The methodology attempted to allow these perspectives to emerge.

The six respondents were each interviewed once, with the interviews lasting approximately one hour. The interviews were carried out between July 1992 and July 1993. Two were carried out in the respondent's home and four at the addiction project, in counselling rooms. Confidentiality was assured, in that no client could be identified from the study data. No comments which might compromise an individual with the agency were reported in a way which might enable that individual to be identified. The interviews were open-ended, and taped for transcription.

Though a basic interview guide was used, the interviews evolved from respondent to respondent, as themes related to disulfiram use became apparent. For example, the theme of **flexible** use of disulfiram, discussed later in the chapter, emerged in early interviews and was actively pursued as more interviews were conducted.

DATA ANALYSIS AND THE EMERGENT MODEL

Introduction

Data was analysed through a combination of the mapping techniques employed by Plummer (1976) for life histories and through a more direct process of coding verbatim transcriptions of users' views on taking disulfiram.

A 'transcript map' was made from each tape. Transcript mapping is a technique of plotting on to paper sequences, processes, biographical information and ideas associated with a life history. The maps allowed the researcher to locate disulfiram users in a time frame, exploring their retrospective accounts of the ways in which the meaning of disulfiram use changed over time.

This method aids analysis in a number of ways. Once mapped, only areas of current interest need be focused upon and fully transcribed. The process allows an interview to be represented visually and quickly scanned when needed. If all interviews are given similar treatment, several maps can be scanned almost simultaneously, allowing identification of potential themes.

Strauss and Corbin (1990) provide a systematic framework for the analysis of qualitative data. They describe three stages of data analysis, involving **open**, **axial** and **selective coding**. These coding techniques are now briefly described in terms of their use in this study.

During open coding, the researcher identifies different themes, and uses them to categorize the data. Four principal themes were identified from the transcript maps at this stage:

- **knowledge/information factors** – variations in user information and knowledge about alcohol, health and disulfiram;
- **abstinence management skills** – skills called upon by users to maintain abstinence in situations of high risk;
- **intrapersonal factors** – processes within an individual such as beliefs, self-image and self-esteem linked with personal use of disulfiram;
- **interpersonal factors** – processes between the disulfiram user and others (family, friends, professionals).

During axial and selective coding, data which has been fractured by open coding is put back together in new ways, illustrative of the interplay between the categories described. Axial coding (Strauss and Corbin, 1990, p. 96) involves focusing on the properties of each principal category identified in open coding, e.g. variations around a theme, relationships to other categories. Selective coding (Strauss and Corbin, 1990, p. 116) is used to fit the principal categories together around a core category, so as to tell a 'story' about the data. Strauss and Corbin (1990, p. 117) emphasize that axial and selective coding cannot be sharply differentiated.

The core category: commitment to abstinence

Well Antabuse is the only thing that's helped me stop drinking. I've tried nearly everything else. (R6)

This quotation illustrates the role of disulfiram in assisting the respondent to achieve the goal of abstinence. Since this goal underpinned the use of disulfiram and linked the categories in a meaningful way, the core category became 'commitment to abstinence'. A model based on this core category is presented in Figure 9.1.

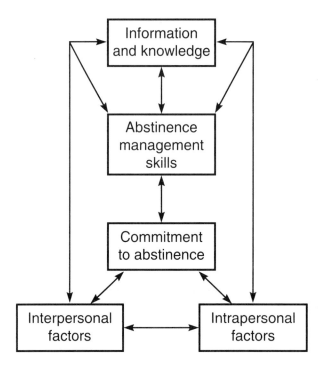

Figure 9.1 A model of commitment to abstinence.

A disulfiram user's commitment to abstinence is governed by the complex interplay between processes identified in the above model. The user is caught up in a web of relationships, and is offered different opinions, advice, information and forms of support. The interplay between categories within the above model can be seen as having a direct bearing on the ways in which different users approach their commitment to abstinence. For example, when a health professional gives information to a client, we see an interplay between the interpersonal and knowledge/information categories, whereas counselling illustrates an interplay between the interpersonal and intrapersonal categories.

Strauss and Corbin (1990) stress the importance of developing the properties and dimensions of categories in order to produce a rich grounded theory. Properties are seldom 'black and white' in terms of dimensions. They usually lie within a continuum of values.

Commitment to abstinence varied both in degree (high versus low) and duration (long versus short). User perspectives on disulfiram can be understood in terms of variations in these dimensions of commitment to abstinence. For example the flexible use of disulfiram discussed below combined a high commitment to abstinence with relatively short duration.

User perspectives on disulfiram

User perspectives on disulfiram will now be considered in more detail, using the categories identified in the abstinence commitment model.

Initiation into disulfiram use

Disulfiram is not always instigated solely by professionals. Other disulfiram-using peers can be a source of information.

> It's been discussed, like, talked about around the table. People, some people, didn't know anything about it until the likes of us talked about it. They asked us what it was about, like. (R1)

Disulfiram is inevitably seen as a 'severe' strategy.

> I said, 'Oh, that's your drinking days finished when you're on that stuff'. It's like part of your life, isn't it? (R3)

Clients could take the very offer of disulfiram as an indicator that their problems were serious.

> After I first talked about Antabuse, I think I realized that I had a very serious drink problem. (R1)

The following quotation is an example of the opposite process, with refusal of disulfiram being taken as a sign that the problem was not severe. More generally, it is a good illustration of the misunderstandings which can arise when patients interpret medical advice from their own perspectives.

> The GP says he wouldn't prescribe it, says 'I don't believe in giving you that.'... He's telling me to stop drinking altogether. I ask for stuff, and he says, 'No I won't give you it'. So I says, 'It can't be that important.' My father says, 'You can't be that bad, then.' (R3)

In this example, the respondent and his father misinterpret the GP's communication. The GP refused disulfiram on therapeutic grounds, but his refusal was seen as an indicator that the alcohol problem was not 'really' serious. The drinker's assessment of his problem is interpersonally mediated, with the father reinforcing his misunderstanding of the medical perspective. The example also illustrates the importance of health professional interpretations of client needs in the new NHS 'internal market' which does not give users any degree of direct choice over the treatments which they receive (Chapter 1).

Who, if anyone, gives clients information about disulfiram, what they understand by the treatment and the views of health professionals, both about its value and individual suitability, are important predisposing factors in the initial take-up of treatment. Negative views of the treatment may well create an ambivalence in the user, which in turn prejudices their chances of staying with it.

Abstinence management skills and high-risk situations

Clients saw disulfiram use as part of a package of adjustment to non-drinking that included the development of abstinence management techniques, ways of coping with high-risk situations and methods for restructuring time.

On first beginning to use disulfiram, individuals may feel uncomfortable in situations seen as high risk. The following quotation concerns exposure to a previous drinking situation by an individual newly prescribed disulfiram.

> It was awful. I tried a couple of oranges. I said, 'Oh, I'm going home, out of the road of this'. You know, the temptation was getting to me. (R3)

However, with repeated exposure and practice, skills in managing high-risk situations may become more developed. The following extract illustrates how a respondent began to learn to deal with anger in different ways.

> Well I can't sort of storm off and say, 'Right, I'm going to the pub and that', so I tend to stop arguing, maybe, in a sense, not really speak to anybody, and sort of cool myself down, and stop the pressure building up. (R2)

At an everyday level, disulfiram operated as a fairly simple barrier, removing the possibility of drinking in response to the temptation.

> Fancying a drink is actually the same. The difference is knowing I'm on Antabuse, I can't drink, so I'll have a tonic water or soft drink. (R2)

Disulfiram was often seen as a back-up, supporting commitment to abstinence.

> So I gave it a go, knowing it was, like, a back-up to keep me off the drink. (R1)

Individuals who were not using disulfiram currently could see it as a future option, should they relapse. Disulfiram thus supported their current commitment.

> But you know that it's there. If I want it, I can see the doctor, and he'll give me it straight away. He'll put me straight back on it 'cause he knows how well I did with it. You know, you can always go back to it if you want. (R5)

Other strategies may be combined with disulfiram to create barriers to anticipated temptations in high-risk situations. In the example below the responsibility of driving a car is involved.

> Well I still go out. So, if I'm out and I fancy a drink I just say 'I can't' to myself. And I know I can't because, apart from being on Antabuse, I'm also taking the car now. So I know I can't risk it. The car stops me as well. (R2)

Some respondents felt that they needed to learn other abstinence management skills, in order to structure their time in new ways which did not centre around alcohol consumption.

> I stopped turning out, tried it, stopping in and not going to the boozer and that, but after a couple of days I was demented. I said, 'I'm not doing this', 'cos I had no other hobbies or nowt. (R3)

Thus, disulfiram users can develop abstinence management skills, while using disulfiram as a back-up in situations of high risk. The very option of disulfiram use can itself be considered as a back-up strategy. Since boredom and lack of viable alternatives to alcohol constitute significant risks, it is important for the problem drinker to structure time productively and adopt other coping/adaptive strategies which can coexist with disulfiram treatment.

Intrapersonal factors

Respondents' management of drinking and abstinence, their self-esteem and their interpersonal relationships were inter-related. Drinking could be seen as a response to psychological distress.

> Oh yes, as soon as I used to get depressed or anything, that's when it started, the drinking. (R5)

The following extract sums up a negative cycle of emotions and drinking behaviour.

> You go out for a drink. You might have four or five pints, and you feel on top of the world. Then you get another one, and you start going down. You start feeling depressed and guilty because you're drinking. The more depressed and guilty you feel, the more you drink, so you end up ratted. That's when you're at risk. (R5)

Perceived loss of control was one of the main elements in this negative cycle.

> It was after a while, when I knew I couldn't control myself. (R4)

However, the emotions involved in drinking were not always negative.

You know how you do something, and you're really proud of it, and you finish work, and you've done a really good job, and things like that. It's like giving yourself a reward if you like. You feel like going for a drink as a reward for your efforts that you've done that day. (R6)

Following the development of commitment to abstinence, the possibility of relapse could be seen as a threat to self-esteem as well as to interpersonal relationships. The following comment is concerned with a hypothetical relapse.

I think I would feel awful really, you know, 'cos all this help that I've gotten.... For one daft binge I've thrown it all away. (R3)

Successful use of disulfiram was not merely a 'technical fix' (Chapter 2), but depended on clients' acceptance of responsibility and belief in its efficacy. The client quoted below associated a more positive outcome of disulfiram use, at the second attempt, with acceptance of responsibility for abstinence.

We talked about it. I said, 'I've tried it before, and it didn't work'. Well, I didn't make it work, like. (R1)

The way in which disulfiram can help to take the conflict out of situations of high risk is illustrated in the following comment.

I think it's a good thing because there's a lot of situations whereby you'd like to walk in a place, and it takes that sort of 'Should I?/shouldn't I?' out of the situation. (R6)

Finally, belief in the strength of the disulfiram/alcohol reaction is an important consideration. The following comment illustrates the importance of assessing the need for a tolerance test on an individual basis.

I was going to have one, but when I seen the state of the video [of a tolerance test], I said, there's no problem. I know what Antabuse entails, so I said it wasn't necessary, you know. (R1)

It is important to consider those factors which are internal to an individual, in terms both of how a strategy such as disulfiram will influence him/her and of the need for other therapeutic interventions such as counselling. This provides a link to the next category.

Interpersonal factors

Users valued interpersonal forms of support which backed up disulfiram, seeing the drug in the context of other treatments.

The Dry Club means a lot to me, tied in with Antabuse and the backing I'm getting from counselling. Well, I'm not getting counselling now, but I know I can if need be. (R1)

Interpersonal contact with a therapist or agency could hold different degrees of importance at different times.

Well, I think it's very significant because I know if I had a relapse or something was going wrong I could always contact.... And I find it quite beneficial to have a chat every now and again, once a week for me, you know. (R6)

Friendships and work relationships could support commitment to abstinence.

My friends know I'm on it, so there's no pressure about having a drink off them, so I feel a lot better in myself, a lot more relaxed. (R2)

I've lost several jobs through alcohol, not because of my ability, but unreliable for going to work and not stopping there. But since I started taking Antabuse I've been, well, respected a lot more at work which I think is good. (R6)

But social influences could also threaten commitment to abstinence, creating situations of high risk.

Quite a few lads I've drank with, 'Oh, away, have a pint', you know. I just say no, but there is just that little bit saying, 'I wonder what it would be like if I wasn't on Antabuse, and I could get drinking with the lads again?' (R1)

Disulfiram use impacted on family relationships in various ways. The following extract illustrates the initial effect of a wife's attempts to 'police' her husband's drinking.

Made me feel a bit like a schoolboy, in a sense where, 'You can't do that'. Sometimes I rebelled against it. In other words, could have led to having a drink secretly. (R2)

However, he came to terms with being supervised by his wife.

Well in a way I'm glad because it's so easy. Like, OK, you might take them for a while, but, OK, I'm on them, I'm doing OK. Then, after a few weeks, try my own will power. So being supervised, she knows I'm taking the tablets. So, in a way, I'm glad because it gives me an incentive to take the tablets. (R2)

Disulfiram use could help to reverse the loss of trust associated with lying about drinking behaviour.

It's also saving me a lot of problems at home because I can stop off anywhere on the way home, and I'm not getting accused of going for a sly drink, where, before, if I was late getting home it was 'You've been drinking!' Where, now I'm on Antabuse, if I'm late I can't get accused of drinking because I can't drink. (R2)

Commitment to abstinence and the use of a medical treatment to control behaviour cannot be divorced from their interpersonal context. This context includes peer support for abstinence or drinking and alternative sources of self-esteem such as work and family relationships.

Disulfiram and commitment to abstinence

The ambivalence which problem drinkers often express about their alcohol use is illustrated in the next quotation.

I wanted to abstain to get my affairs sorted out. But I can't explain how I felt at the time. I was frightened to abstain. (R1)

However, once a commitment to abstinence has been made, disulfiram users have some clear ideas about how disulfiram assists their ongoing efforts to abstain.

The seven days before alcohol can be ingested is a recurrent theme, as illustrated in the following comment, concerning taking a disulfiram tablet.

Here's another week before I can have a drink, breathing space. (R4)

Clients made comparisons that helped them to think about their use of disulfiram.

Well I sort of, I've been taking Antabuse for a while now, and I think it's something like having savings in the bank. You can walk about the streets with no money in your pocket with the assurance that there's money in the bank if you need it, you know. (R6)

In this comparison, 'savings' represent alcohol, and the seven day wait equates to 'notice of withdrawal'.

Flexible use of disulfiram

The following extracts are taken from disulfiram users who have used disulfiram in a more flexible way, often negotiating with spouse, family and/or therapist to cease and then recommence disulfiram use at specific times. Special occasions were often involved.

As I say, if a special occasion comes up, like my birthday, and I was drinking for three days, fourth day, drying out. Now I look at it, I find it easier to come on Antabuse because I know what I've spent in them three days was a waste of money. But I'd planned it, so it's up to me. (R1)

These episodes could be incorporated within a commitment to abstinence because they were planned and had a clear end point.

It meant that I'd planned for this. It was like saving up for a holiday.... But I knew that at the end of it I'd have to go back on the Antabuse again, which I did. I can remember thinking, 'When's my next little window? When should I do that?' (R6)

The quantities of alcohol involved may be large.

I enjoy it at the time, but the first day and maybe half the second day I have a good drink, and I mean a bloody good drink. (R1)

However, the above respondent was confident that, through disulfiram, he could re-establish control over his drinking.

I can plan these things because I know at the end of this binge, or celebration, or whatever I've got Antabuse to back me up, and that's very important to me. (R1)

Flexible use of disulfiram enabled these respondents to establish a sense of control over their drinking. Disulfiram thus provided these users with what was, for them, an optimum solution to the 'wicked problem' of drinking, since they could enjoy some drinking bouts without losing control over the longer term. However, this view was not always appreciated by prescribers, therapists and supporting agencies.

When I came off it, [past helper] was a bit upset, not upset, disappointed, well, by his manner and the way he was talking to me. (R1)

The core requirements of a therapeutic relationship have been described by various popular therapists (e.g. Egan, 1986) as genuineness, empathy and respect. Respect involves not judging a client. It may be counter-productive to add to clients' existing self-doubts by expressing negative opinions of their plans.

DISCUSSION

The model of commitment to abstinence developed in this study (Figure 9.1) is based upon the complexities of clients' own perspectives on their needs. Disulfiram use has to be understood in the context of the client's intrapersonal processes (e.g. loss of self-esteem arising from loss of control over drinking) and interpersonal relationships (e.g. restoring trust lost through a history of lying about drinking behaviour).

Previous research into disulfiram has been concerned with measuring outcomes, and has inevitably involved a reductionist, quantitative approach (Brewer, 1986; Critchfield and Eddy, 1987). However, this approach does not consider the meaning of successful or unsuccessful use of disulfiram.

The present research complements these findings by exploring the perspectives of clients who have found the drug useful. Clients who used disulfiram flexibly would not meet the criterion of abstaining for a year used by Critchfield and Eddy (1987), but felt that flexible use enabled them to enjoy limited, controlled drinking bouts. They were thus able to take a medically oriented technical fix designed to control their behaviour, and manage it to meet their own ends.

The study data suggest that disulfiram therapy can be helpful to clients in the following ways:

- providing a 'breathing space' within which underlying problems can be addressed, and new skills learned and practised;
- providing a safety margin when commitment to abstinence fluctuates. Abstinence thus continues, behaviourally speaking, during the fluctuation of commitment;
- providing a back-up to the individual's abstinence management skills.

The use of disulfiram raises issues about client access and medical control. Instead of being offered an option like disulfiram on the basis of prognostic selection criteria and fixed patterns of agreed use, clients could be given information and invited to explore effective use in their own personal contexts. They would be invited to make an informed choice about trying out the treatment and about developing a pattern of use adapted to their own needs and circumstances.

CHAPTER 10

How adults with learning difficulties and their carers see 'the community'

Bob Heyman and Sarah Huckle

INTRODUCTION

This chapter discusses some results from a qualitative study of the perspectives of adults with learning difficulties (adults) attending adult training centres (ATCs) and their carers. Fieldwork, which began in 1991, was carried out with 20 adults, their main informal carers and eight formal carers at the ATCs. In 1993, seven adults and informal carers were re-interviewed, to explore their views of the findings and any changes since the first interviews. Data analysis has revolved around the 'core construct' (Strauss and Corbin, 1990, p. 116) of hazard management (Heyman and Huckle, 1993a, b).

A model of the strategies which adults and informal carers used to manage hazards will be presented. Applying this model, we will consider adults' sense of locality, their developmental status and the ATC as a community. This analysis will be used to raise questions about the future role of ATCs.

BACKGROUND

The concept of learning difficulty

There are problems both in determining the criteria that should be used to classify people as having a particular type of disability and in deciding what label to apply to such people. For our research purposes, we will treat 'adult with learning difficulty' as a description of a social status, in this case defined by attendance at an ATC. It is not assumed that adults had a common underlying disability.

The concept of 'mental handicap', now out of favour, focused attention on to presumed biological impairments of the individual which cause intellectual deficiencies and was thus consistent with the medical model. Since the 1980s the terms 'learning disability' and 'learning difficulty' have come to be favoured in the UK academic and professional literature. Describing people as 'mentally handicapped' has been shown to be more stigmatizing than describing them as having a 'learning difficulty', for example evoking unfavourable stereotypes (Eayrs, Ellis and Jones, 1993). A focus on 'learning' has the advantage of drawing attention to the distinction between potential and attainment, implying that 'sufferers' can learn if appropriate strategies are adopted. The change in terminology is thus part of a wider shift from a medical to a social management model of health problems, as discussed in Chapter 2.

The terms 'learning difficulty' and 'learning disability' have different nuances. 'Learning disability' tends to be preferred in the health literature and reflects a medical tradition, even if an attempt is being made to get away from a purely medical model (e.g. Felce, Taylor and Wright, 1992). 'Disability' locates the 'problem' within the person presumed to be disabled, but a 'learning' disability is implicitly open to amelioration through 'training'.

'Learning difficulty' is more likely to be used in the sociological literature, e.g. in the journal *Disability, Handicap and Society* (to be renamed *Disability and Society* from 1994). The term is neutral, at least in theory, about the location of the difficulty. A learning difficulty may be caused by the students and/or the teachers (in a broad sense). For example, adults may fail to learn not because of cognitive disability but because they are not allowed to develop or practise certain skills, e.g. locality navigation, forming sexual relationships. Disability must be reconstructed as a social response to individual problems (Oliver, 1992).

There is evidence that adults living with their parents are prevented from developing everyday living skills at home (Flynn and Saleem, 1986) and that parents often underestimate their abilities (Block, 1980) and interpersonal needs (Richardson and Ritchie, 1989). Research into adults' family relationships has sometimes had an unfortunate parent-blaming tone. It obscures the rational basis in danger avoidance of apparent parental 'overprotectiveness' (Heyman and Huckle, 1993b). Nevertheless, this research does suggest that learning difficulty arises from limits in learning opportunities as well as cognitive disabilities.

It should not be assumed that lay usage corresponds to that of academics and professionals. The informal carers in our research tended to favour the more global term 'handicapped' without the 'mental', while most adults with learning difficulties strongly resisted the idea that they were 'handicapped', at least in research interviews. Neither adults nor informal carers used the term 'learning difficulty', and the adults did not understand what it meant.

Normalization

A social management approach to a health problem requires a strong consensus about the aims of intervention. During the 1980s, in Britain and other countries, attempts were made to develop such a consensus around the goal of normalization for people with learning difficulties (Whitehead, 1992). The concepts of learning difficulty and normalization are interconnected in that one of the main methods for achieving normalization is training in everyday living skills. To be worth attempting, this strategy requires an assumption that persons with learning difficulties are capable of learning such skills. As will be illustrated below, informal carers often do not accept this assumption.

The concepts of learning difficulty and normalization both direct attention away from value issues. 'Learning difficulty' begs questions about what people with varying capabilities ought to learn while 'normalization' raises a host of issues concerning what is normal and whether normality is good. The problem of defining what is normal in specific contexts is ignored and the ways in which individuals actively construct normality are obscured (Heyman and Huckle, 1993a). In our research, we have found that an activity such as the adult moving freely about the locality or having a sexual relationship could be seen as normal or abnormal depending upon the observer's framework (danger avoidance, limited or extended risk taking).

Policies which are blind to adults and informal carers' own belief systems are doomed to fail because they are almost certain to provoke negative reactions which policy makers and practitioners fail to understand (Cattermole, Jahoda and Markova, 1987). The response of some adults with learning difficulties and their informal carers to community care policies can be understood as resistance to what they see as enforced normalization. Attempts to focus on individual choice in service provision (O'Brien, 1987) are part of a wider shift from a social management to a consumerist model of care, discussed in Chapter 2.

METHODOLOGY

Introduction

Research into client perspectives can help policy makers and practitioners to take a more anthropological approach to service users. However, research must attempt to do justice to the complexities of the views which real people hold, a challenging task. The adults we spoke to were constantly subject to the dual authority of formal and informal carers, and lived in fear of 'getting wrong'. They inevitably tended to tell the interviewer what they thought she wanted to hear. It was necessary to talk to adults at length over several sessions, to develop relationships of trust and to carefully sift the evidence from the entire interview in order to arrive at a judgement, inevitably subjective, about what adults 'really' thought. Adult views have to be put into the context of those of informal carers. We need to do justice to a diversity of opinions as well as looking for patterns and similarities.

There can be no guarantee that the right conclusions have been drawn from this inescapably qualitative process although we have adopted the procedure, usual in qualitative research, of feeding back our conclusions to adults, informal and formal carers and asking them if we have got things right.

The sample

Our initial aim was to investigate the needs of young adults with learning difficulties who had lived from birth with informal carers (usually parents) in the community. The research aims thus excluded adults who had been 'decanted' out of long-stay hospitals as a result of community care reforms during the 1980s.

The scope of the research rapidly narrowed, for purely pragmatic reasons, and was confined to adults attending two ATCs who had sufficient communication ability to participate in a simple interview and who were therefore in the upper ability range. The ATCs were located in an urban area of Tyne and Wear characterized by high levels of poverty and unemployment but also substantial pockets of affluence. The final sample contained a social mix of families with professional, skilled manual and manual social backgrounds, with varying employment status and income levels.

Narrowing the scope of the research eased data collection. It would have been difficult to obtain a reliable list of adults with learning difficulties living in the community and the definitional problems seemed awesome. The price paid was that some interesting groups were excluded from the research, for example adults whose informal carers had kept them out of the segregated environment of the ATC. These excluded informal carers are likely to have been more positive towards normalization than those whom we interviewed.

Although the decision to focus on relatively accomplished adults at ATCs was taken pragmatically, the group selected turned out to be theoretically interesting. As the most capable attenders at the ATC, their membership was marginal. Depending upon how their potential abilities were viewed, these adults could be seen as needing the protective environment of the ATC or as capable of a less sheltered life. Because the adults were marginal relative to the institution of the ATC, conflicts in interpretations of their potential for normalization were easily detectable.

The main sample consisted of 20 adults (10 male and 10 female) drawn from the two ATCs. At least one informal carer of each adult was interviewed, as were eight formal carers at the two ATCs. In 1993, two years after the initial interviews, seven adults and their main informal carers were re-interviewed. These families were 'theoretically sampled' (Strauss and Corbin, 1990, p. 176) in order to explore different approaches to managing hazards. One family was chosen because it appeared to have 'flipped' from danger avoidance to limited risk taking between the first and the second interview.

The refusal rate was minimal, perhaps because the interviewer (SH) attended the ATCs informally on several occasions before interviewing commenced, perhaps because the adults were a 'captive audience'. All 20 adults and informal carers agreed to participate in the first interviews, as did the eight formal carers. One informal carer refused to take part in the second interview because she felt that she had 'had enough' of the research.

Methods

Interviews with adults, which were private and confidential, took place over several sessions at the ATC and lasted six to nine hours in total.

Interviewing was semi-structured. The researcher asked a series of general questions covering leisure, work and the ATC, education, friendships, opposite sex relationships, home life and future prospects. Open-ended questions were asked to minimize acquiescence (Sigelman *et al.*, 1981), and then progressively focused if necessary.

Interviews with informal carers were conducted at home in a single session, and took three to six hours to complete. These interviews mainly covered their views of the adult's prospects in the areas mentioned above and their views of the adult's views (i.e. their metaperspectives, as discussed in Chapter 1). Formal carers were interviewed at the ATC about the adults' potential and need for independence and about relationships between formal and informal carers. These interviews were carried out after extensive analysis of adult and informal carer interviews. They were informed by the major theme which emerged, coping with hazards, as discussed below.

The second-stage interviews were relatively short (30–60 minutes), and were, again, conducted privately and confidentially, at the ATC for adults and at home for informal carers. These interviews focused on two areas: discussion of a brief report describing the main findings of the research (explained verbally to adults); and any significant changes which had occurred since the first interviews.

Data analysis

All interviews were taped and fully transcribed into computerized word-processor files. Full transcription, which is time-consuming, is not always recommended. (An alternative approach based on 'transcript mapping' and selective transcription was used in the research into alcohol problems discussed in Chapter 9.)

Our analysis, which has gone on for over two years, was initially based on detailed consideration of four of the 20 cases. It was then extended to other cases in order to see if patterns were repeated. We were eventually using all 20 cases, and this led to some quantitative analysis, introduced below. Although we did not initially use the full data set, we were eventually glad that all the tapes had been transcribed (by SH) in the early, most enthusiastic stages of the research. Interviewing, transcription and preliminary analysis were carried out concurrently. This was useful for identifying problems in interviewing technique, e.g. inadvertently leading questions and areas which needed further clarification. For example, adults and informal carers were often vague about how often the adult saw friends outside the ATC. The interviewer learnt to gently probe this sensitive topic in order to obtain more specific information.

The stages of qualitative analysis corresponded roughly to those proposed by Strauss and Corbin (1990). In the first stage, 'open coding', four adult and informal carer transcripts were cut up, and sorted according to a variety of emergent themes (using the database within WordPerfect). The interviews covered a range of topics (see above). At this stage, the researchers experienced considerable anxiety through not having a clear direction.

Fortunately, a direction quickly emerged. We were struck by the extent to which adult and informal carer accounts of the adults' lives were dominated by the need to cope with the perceived hazards of 'normal life'.

The emergent theme of coping with hazards provided the basis for the second stage identified by Strauss and Corbin (1990), that of 'axial coding'. At this stage, the properties of categories that have emerged during open coding are explored. Our key to axial coding was the observation that adults and informal carers coped with hazards in two distinct ways, either as risks to be calculated or as dangers to be avoided (discussed further below). Although most adults and informal carers used both methods for dealing with hazards, it was apparent that risk taking was tolerated more by some families than by others.

We were then able to make connections between risk taking/danger avoidance and other categories. Quantification through coding of qualitative data (Silverman, 1985) was used to assess relationships which were identified. For example, adults from more risk-tolerant families were judged by formal carers at the ATCs to be achieving more of their potential (Heyman and Huckle, 1993b).

The third stage of qualitative analysis identified by Strauss and Corbin (1990) is 'selective coding'. In this stage, which cannot be clearly distinguished from axial coding, the relationships that have been identified during selective coding are elaborated into a 'story' concerning the tactics and strategies which people adopt to deal with perceived problems. This

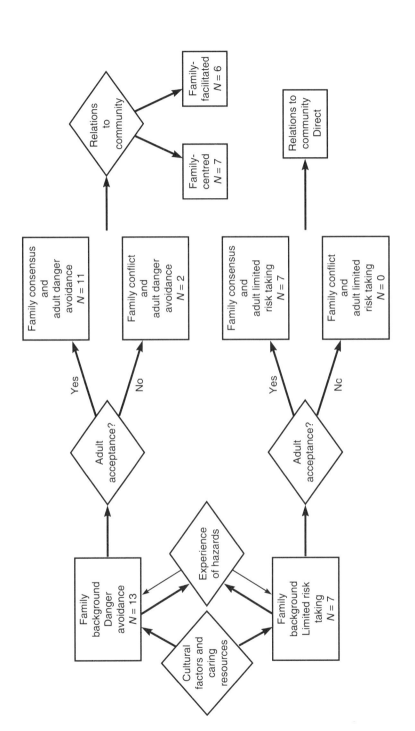

Figure 10.1 Adults with learning difficulties – family background, experience and hazards ($n = 20$)

'story' is mapped in Figure 10.1, and is applied to adults' relationships with the community in the Results section of this chapter.

RESULTS

Managing hazards

We will use 'hazard' as a neutral term to describe an action or situation which is perceived to have a probability, however small, of negative outcomes. The observer may categorize a hazard as a risk or a danger. Risks may be calculated, minimized and subject to cost–benefit analysis. They may be taken or not taken in particular circumstances. Dangers should be avoided. The same hazard, e.g. the adult going out alone, may be seen by different observers as a risk or a danger.

Hazards pose a 'wicked problem' for groups perceived as vulnerable, including those with learning difficulties, because strategies that maximize their autonomy (e.g. allowing them to move freely around the locality) expose them to hazards while a 'safety first' approach restricts their autonomy. The model presented in Figure 10.1 attempts to map the strategies adopted by adults and informal carers to manage this wicked problem. The main elements and interactions in the model are summarized below.

Cultural factors and caring resources

The ways in which families managed hazards were closely related to their social circumstances. More prosperous families and those which had both parents as informal carers (closely overlapping groups) were markedly more likely to treat hazards as dangers to be avoided. One explanation of this finding is that these families had more 'caring resources' and so were better able to protect adults from perceived danger, ironically with negative results in terms of their integration with the wider community. Another explanation, perhaps related, is that families with lower socioeconomic status were culturally more accepting of an adult with learning difficulties (Carr, 1975).

Family background: danger avoidance

The informal carers in 13 families had a 'safety first' approach and treated perceived hazards primarily as dangers to be avoided. Living independently, marriage, sexual relationships, getting a job outside the ATC and moving freely around the locality were all considered unsafe and beyond the adults' capabilities, even with 'training'. The adults in these families, on the whole, shared this danger avoidance perspective. However, there were two 'rebels' and others showed less obvious signs of frustration with the constraints associated with danger avoidance.

Family background: limited risk taking

A second group of seven families were almost equally pessimistic about the adult's ability to live independently, get married, etc. but were willing, with considerable anxiety and safeguards, to give him/her partial freedom of the locality. As a result, these adults were able to develop their own lives outside the family and the ATC, for example to visit friends and relatives independently, to maintain a private relationship with a member of the opposite sex (despite the risk, from informal carer perspectives, of sexual activity) or to become established at local pubs and clubs.

Experience

The experiences which adults and informal carers had with hazards, either directly or reported indirectly, were coloured by their implicit 'theories' about risks and dangers. Because hazards are intangible, experiences could always be used or selected to confirm a preferred view.

Interviewer: Why shouldn't you talk to strangers?

Adult: I might get mugged, hurt, abused, take me away in a car. I might also get run down by a car. That is why my dad helps me cross the road for the bus every morning. (Adult F1)

One adult, according to a formal carer, had been trained to travel locally but was stopped from doing this by her parents when she stepped in front of a car. The formal carer pointed out that many 'normal' people become involved in traffic incidents without questions being raised about their underlying competence. The parents were not merely responding to 'evidence', but actively fitting contingencies into a framework based on the assumption of unavoidable adult vulnerability.

Accounts of experiences which changed adult or informal carer perspectives on hazards were much rarer than accounts of experiences which confirmed them. One informal carer who allowed 'his' adult to move around the locality relatively freely had stopped her from going to the local pub on her own after a man tried to molest her, even though the locals had intervened and given the man 'a good hiding'.

Adults who were allowed to take limited risks were subject to contingencies (e.g. getting lost or attacked) which, if they occurred, were likely to lead to a more restrictive regime, through being taken as evidence of the inherent dangerousness of the activity in question. If adults were not allowed to undertake an activity because it was considered too dangerous, direct evidence about contingencies was cut off and there was no way to learn that the activity (perhaps) was acceptably safe.

For this reason, examples of deciding that contingencies previously considered dangerous were safe were rare. The example given below, from the Stage Two interviews, concerns the one family that 'flipped' from danger avoidance to limited risk taking. The change was associated with formal carers persuading the adult's mother to allow him to make journeys on his own, under carefully controlled conditions. Having experienced these as safe, she became more willing to extend his zone of autonomy.

> **Interviewer**: Do you let [adult] go to Newcastle on the bus on his own?
>
> **Informal carer**: Yes it was the other day. It has taken me all these years to finally let him do it. I was worried stiff. I didn't think he was on the bus. I met him at the other end you see.
>
> **Interviewer**: Will you let him do it again?
>
> **Informal carer**: Yes I think so. He seemed to manage all right, but you can't help being protective can you? (Adult M8)

Adult acceptance

In general, adults' reported perspectives on hazards corresponded closely to those of their informal carers. For example, adults were more likely to mention dangers frequently in interview if their informal carers did so (Heyman and Huckle, 1993b). Given the power that informal carers had, it is reasonable to assume that adults acquired their attitudes to risks and dangers from them. However, the adults did not just passively accept informal carer perspectives. A number of adults in families oriented towards danger avoidance expressed frustration about lives largely restricted to the ATC and family. These frustrations tended to surface only after the interviewer had known the adults for some time. Two adults, both male, actively rebelled against these restrictions, as noted above, seeking to marry, live independently and get jobs.

Family consensus and adult risk taking

In theory, four outcomes were possible within the framework we have developed. Informal carers could encourage or discourage adults from taking limited risks and adults could accept or reject the strategy offered for managing hazards. The number of families in which each of these four outcomes was found is shown in Figure 10.1. There were no families in this sample in which adults were pressured, against their wishes, into taking risks.

One of the two adults classified as a rebel in the Stage One interviews was re-interviewed and seemed more accepting, or resigned, two years later.

Interviewer: Do you ever still think about leaving the centre?

Adult: No, I am quite sorted, and I am quite happy with what I do. I shut up now. I can't change anything. Mam won't listen. It causes too much trouble, so I don't say anything. (Adult M1)

Community relations

Adults in families that tolerated limited risks were able to undertake their own activities, independently of carers and to develop direct, but limited, relationships to the wider community. One adult was known in his local pub and visited members of his extended family. One went to local non-segregated clubs with a boyfriend who also had learning difficulties. Another 'played' with local companions. All the limited risk takers were able to visit friends from the ATC on their own and to engage in independent activities in the locality, e.g. going to the town centre.

Adults in families which managed hazards primarily through danger avoidance could only interact with the wider community under the protection of carers. These families had the secondary problem of managing adults' leisure time and adopted one of two strategies to do this. Some informal carers facilitated adult activities, for example participating actively in clubs for adults with learning difficulties and escorting them on trips and holidays. The adult became a 'project', giving meaning to informal carers' lives. Through facilitated activities, the adult could enjoy a varied life without being exposed to danger. The inevitable price was paid in terms of adult autonomy, since their activities were essentially determined and controlled by their informal carers.

Informal carer: Well I would say if [adult] was in the house instead of going out [adult] would talk and talk ... so I would rather take him out. It gets me out as well, and I can meet the parents, which I enjoy. (Adult M4)

The alternative strategy was for families to define the adult's needs as essentially filled through a life revolving round the ATC and family-centred activities.

Informal carer: I think she comes home from work [ATC] tired and, in our terms, she is a bit overweight. She is glad of a sit down when she comes in. She doesn't want to go and do anything very physical any more. (Adult F3)

The adult referred to was not so happy with this restricted definition of her needs.

Interviewer: Would you like to see your friends more on an evening?

Adult: Yes, I would like to see [adults from ATC] But I don't have a chance to see [adult]. (Adult F3)

The next part of the chapter will discuss the themes which emerged from our data concerning the degree of adult integration into the wider local community. These themes were: adults' varying 'cognitive maps' of their locality; the ambiguous developmental status attributed to some adults by carers; the different ways in which the family mediated between adults and the wider community; and the role of the ATC as a community.

Community integration

Adults' cognitive maps of the locality

Adults from danger-avoiding families appeared to magnify distances, so that space which would be experienced as local and familiar by 'normal' people was felt to be far away.

Interviewer: Is [adult friend at ATC] able to visit your home?

Adult: No, he lives too far away. (Adult M6)

The friend referred to lived two to three miles away.

Adults from these families often expressed a fear of getting lost, frequently mentioned as a barrier to developing greater mobility skills.

Interviewer: Do you ever go to his house?

Adult: No, because I don't know where he lives.

Interviewer: Would you like to call to his house?

Adult: No, in case my mum would not let us. I might get lost or something. (Adult M8)

Adults from limited risk-taking families, although by no means free of fear of strangers or of getting lost, experienced the locality as a more familiar, smaller, less threatening place.

Interviewer: Do you think you have enough things to do on a weekend?

Adult: Sometimes I go to my nana's.

Interviewer: Do you walk over?

Adult: On my own. And sometimes I go to my sister's as well.... And my auntie's too.

Interviewer: Do they live near you?

Adult: My sister lives close, but my grandma is further away. [She lived about a mile away]. (Adult M9)

Difficulty in classifying adults' developmental status

Some families had problems classifying adults' developmental status. They felt that the person they were caring for was an adult in some respects (chronological age, length of experience, biological sexuality), but a child in others (understanding, emotional maturity).

> **Informal carer**: Some areas of her mind are very experienced, because she has still experienced 30 years of life.... She has an awful lot of experiences to draw on, and she has a very good memory.... But she still attacks things as a lot of six-year-olds would. (Adult F1)

Such problems were raised only by members of families oriented to danger avoidance, suggesting that adult ambiguous developmental status was associated with living a highly sheltered life. Smooth interaction depends upon a clear, shared definition of the situation and encounters where the definition of the situation is ambiguous or equivocal are particularly difficult to manage (Harré and Secord, 1972). Thus, ambiguous developmental status was a barrier to community integration.

Problems associated with adults' ambiguous developmental status came out particularly clearly in connection with their past and present relationships with other children. In all but one case, adults went through a process of withdrawal from social ties with 'normal' friends as they grew older and the gap between themselves and peers appeared to widen.

Siblings often maintained supportive relationships and, by taking the adult out, provided rare opportunities for adults to engage the local community in the company of their own generation. Occasionally, developmental distancing occurred even with siblings.

> **Interviewer**: Does he see his brother?

> **Informal carer**: About once a year.... Before he started school he got on well with [adult], then when he was five and [adult] was 10 it changed.... I remember his first open night at the school, and he said, 'You won't bring [adult], will you?'. (Adult M6)

In the present, there were sometimes difficulties in otherwise positive relationships between adults and young relatives.

> **Informal carer**: She has a computer.... I think it may well be that what upsets [adult] slightly about it is there are one or two programmes that [adult] can do, while [child], the six-year-old, can do more programs than [adult] can do. (Adult F1)

Adults, particularly those from danger-avoiding families, were acutely sensitive to symbolic denigration of their developmental status.

Adult: They [carers at the ATC] talk to you like you are a baby. (Adult F3)

The social awkwardness associated with ambiguous developmental status, and the resulting barrier to adults participating in the wider community, are illustrated in the next section.

Family and family-mediated relationships

Adults from limited risk-taking families were able to develop some relationships for themselves, while those from danger-avoiding families could only participate in activities organized by carers. Although adults reported that they enjoyed these activities, they had a number of limitations in terms of adult self-expression.

Firstly, the adult was sometimes marginalized in activities designed primarily to meet the needs of informal carers.

Interviewer: What do you do at your nana's?

Adult: They have a talk, and I listen. (Adult F1)

Secondly, informal carers sometimes reported embarrassment at adults' perceived lack of social competence.

Informal carer: She sort of monopolizes the conversation and brings it all down to her level. So it is embarrassing to take her somewhere too often. (Adult F3)

Thirdly, distress and potential conflict arose for both adults and informal carers because of the stigmatizing responses of other members of the community.

Informal carer: I remember one year going to Scarborough, and some people walking past saying, 'What a tragedy'.

Interviewer: What do you think?

Informal carer: Not a lot. (Adult M6)

In contrast, as noted above, adults from limited risk-taking families were able to develop their own independent relationships, with friends from the ATC and, to a lesser extent, other members of the community. The adult quoted below expresses awareness of the qualitative difference between her own relationships and those that are family-mediated.

Interviewer: Would you ever like to go out with them [informal carer and his girlfriend]?

Adult: No, I like them to go by themselves. I don't want to get in the way. My boyfriend takes us to the pub on a weekend.

Interviewer: Do you meet any other friends when you go to the pub?

Adult: Yes. His mate. (Adult F7)

The ATC as a community

Adult perspectives
As discussed in Chapter 1, a 'symbolic community' is a set of people who define themselves as similar to each other and different to non-members in certain respects (Cohen, 1985). However, the similarity defining membership of the ATC was potentially stigmatizing. The adults faced a definitional dilemma. On the one hand, they mostly valued the activities provided by the ATC, for example opportunities for friendship.

Interviewer: Why do you want to stay here [ATC]?

Adult: Because I left school and [boyfriend] is here as well.... I am here with all my friends. (Adult F1)

On the other hand, their membership of this 'community' put them into a symbolically inferior position *vis à vis* non-members.

The adults were asked why they thought they attended the ATC, and whether they thought they were 'handicapped'. There was a hermeneutic problem. The politically correct term 'learning difficulties' was not used or understood by adults or informal carers, and we were forced to use the discredited term 'handicapped'.

When asked directly, the adults mostly rejected the term 'handicapped', although it was used frequently by carers. Most drew a distinction within the ATC between adults, like themselves, and those who were 'really' handicapped because of physical disability.

Adult: We are not mentally handicapped, but special care are.

Interviewer: Why are special care different?

Adult: Because they are in wheelchairs, but we are not in wheelchairs. (Adult M10)

Adults saw the ATC as a place where they worked rather than a place where they learned, a view that avoided stigmatization but obscured the training function of the ATC. The training function was further obscured because adults were rarely able to practise at home skills acquired at the ATC and because of a lack of continuity in training. One adult was mystified by a volunteer's attempt to teach him to use the bus. The quotation illustrates the importance of considering the meaning of interventions from the adult's perspective.

Interviewer: So you did use a bus on your own [with trainer following by car]?

Adult: Yes. I thought a lot about all of that, but he [trainer] didn't come back here again. And every Tuesday, he always comes on a Tuesday. And sometimes I see him and talk to him, but he didn't come back. You won't believe that. That's really true, that. (Adult M10)

Informal carer perspectives

Informal carers valued the ATC highly and resisted suggestions that the adult might move on. One reason for this resistance was informal carers' fear that they might be left with 24-hour responsibility for the adult's lifestyle.

Informal carer: When he was at home for a year, before he went to the centre, I was always taking him to places, letting him do what he wanted to do, playing bandits and things like that, playing pool. I had to. He had nothing else. (Adult M1)

Implicit in this account was the assumption, particularly in danger-avoiding families, that adults could not develop their own independent activities. Therefore, if the ATC was not available, full responsibility would fall on to informal carers, and the quality of adults' lives would suffer.

In relation to normalization, community care can be conceptualized as a series of stages leading to greater independence, for example ATC/sheltered employment/full employment. But, from the perspective of informal carers, such systems could be seen as a one-way escalator, moving away from the ATC.

Informal carer: I wouldn't want him to get a job and then find out he didn't like it, because then he couldn't get his place back at the centre straight away. It took us a year to get [adult] a place in here in the first place. (Adult M1)

This theme of managing a moving escalator of scarce care occurs in other chapters, in the use of sheltered accommodation by the elderly (Chapter 7) and attempts by HIV patients to obtain benefits (Chapter 12).

The quotation below illustrates the way in which some informal carers saw the 'authorities' as pushing vulnerable adults out into a dangerous world without adequate care. It also illustrates the distinction which informal carers made between lay and professional knowledge and commitment.

Informal carer: I think the authority had brought up the issue [sex education] because they were intending for all of them, at some time, to be living out in the community. As much as we don't agree with it, they want to do it, but they would only be willing to put in a certain number of hours of supervision.... Although they can do many things, they need someone there who will give them that kick and push to go on and do those things.... It is all right for the authority saying do this and that, but who is more qualified to say what should be done than the parent who has lived with them for 40 years? (Adult F1)

DISCUSSION

Adults, informal and formal carers had quite different perspectives on adult needs and capabilities. There were substantial differences between families who had danger-avoidance and limited risk-taking approaches to hazard management. Formal carers at the ATCs were strongly pro-risk and felt that most of these adults were capable, variously, of independent or semi-independent living, responsible sexual relationships, marriage and unsheltered employment (Heyman and Huckle, 1993b). Their approach could be described as 'extended risk taking'. Formal carers explained parental caution and desire to keep the adult in the ATC in psychological terms, as overprotective or financially motivated. They failed to see that danger avoidance was, from an informal carer perspective, a rational response to the 'wicked problem' of managing hazards for vulnerable people.

All of the informal carers (but not all the adults) felt that the adults did not have even the potential ability to manage extended risk taking. For them, and for many adults, the ATC was an alternative safe community, providing friendship, recreation and work activities.

The manager of one ATC expressed understandable disappointment that our research report had not mentioned all their hard work to promote normalization through training in everyday living skills. This omission arose because we could only 'see' what respondents told us from their perspectives and training was hardly mentioned. The adults saw themselves as going to the ATC to work, implying a permanent occupation.

Although the adults in our sample all led highly restricted lives, there were marked differences between those living in danger-avoiding and limited risk-taking families. The latter were able to establish independent relationships within the locality while the former saw their locality as an alien, threatening place. Research into the social relationships of stigmatized groups, like that cited at the beginning of this chapter, has tended to stress the sociology of exclusion. It is equally important to analyse the conditions in which those with learning difficulties include themselves, and are included, in the community (Evans and Murcott, 1990).

ATCs have obvious disadvantages in that they segregate adults from the wider community, challenge their self-esteem and promote parent–child relationships between staff and trainees. The large-scale closure of ATCs is now on the agenda, partly in response to the more flexible climate stimulated by the NHS and Community Care Act 1990. However, before ATCs are closed or alternatives developed, their functions need to be carefully considered, particularly for adults who exist physically in a locality but have no meaningful relationship with it.

Community care for adults with learning difficulties, of whatever form, should involve the development of partnerships between adults, informal and formal carers. This will require greater recognition of each other's perspective. There is a danger that, by adopting a pro-risk social management strategy, formal carers will provoke resistance in families and unintentionally reduce the opportunities for adults with learning difficulties to choose to take or not to take risks.

CHAPTER 11

Mental illness in the community: the role of voluntary and state agencies

Elizabeth Handyside and Bob Heyman

INTRODUCTION

The research discussed in this chapter (Handyside, 1989; Handyside and Heyman, 1990) involved an evaluation of the effectiveness of a community mental health scheme. Qualitative and quantitative changes in the mental health of individuals participating in this scheme were compared with those occurring in a control group receiving conventional community mental health services. The chapter also illustrates how qualitative and quantitative methods can be combined.

The chapter begins with a consideration of problems of defining 'mental illness' and 'community mental health care'. The next section discusses the background, aims and methodology of the research. The main quantitative and qualitative results are then presented and discussed.

What is mental illness?

The role of covert value judgements

Despite its commonly assumed meaning, mental illness is particularly difficult to define. Proponents of the medical model assert that mental illness is similar in kind to a physical illness and that treatment should therefore be biomedical, e.g. drug therapies, electroconvulsive shock therapy.

On the other hand, relativists argue that mental illness is defined in relation to culturally specific rather than universal norms. Butler and Pritchard (1983) and Goffman (1971), for example, argue that mental disorder is a social construct depending on the particular norms of each society and the social context in which behaviour may be judged appropriate. Behaviour which might be labelled as mental illness in one culture might be viewed as 'normal' in another. 'Treatment', from this perspective, would involve either changing social norms or teaching individuals to conform to them.

It is logically impossible to make judgements about mental illness without drawing on assumptions, implicit or explicit, about the nature of mental health. And notions of mental health in turn rely on value judgements about 'the good life' which are rarely spelt out explicitly. In the words of Szasz (1970): 'The statement, "X is a mental symptom" involves rendering a judgement that entails a covert comparison between the patient's ideas, concepts and beliefs and those of the observer and the society in which they live' (p. 14). Szasz argues that the term 'illness', when attributed to a mental disorder, is really being used as a metaphor. He suggests that, in the past, doctors treated people who acted strangely as if they were ill. Strange behaviour evolved into 'mental illness'. What people are really suffering from, according to Szasz, are problems of living, not diseases. He therefore argues that mental illness *per se* is a myth. This argument poses a real difficulty for professionals trying to 'treat' such an illness. The accounts which 'mentally ill' people give of their own 'problems of living' were one of the main focuses of the present research.

The power of labels

Proponents of labelling theory (Scheff, 1966) believe that the label 'mentally ill' is sufficient to produce the incomprehensible behaviours and social rejection that are still commonly associated with mental health problems. 'Official labelling can transform a person's beliefs about devaluation and discrimination of mental patients into an expectation of rejection' (Link, 1987, p. 97). This expectation may become a self-proving reality as the labelled individual, his/her family, the professionals and the community all start playing their roles. Being diagnosed as mentally ill may itself be at least part of the 'problem' which community mental health services need to 'treat'.

What is community mental health care?

In Chapter 1, the difficulty of defining 'community health care' was discussed at length. If we add in the problematic concept of mental health/illness, a theoretical definition of community mental health care becomes elusive.

The image of community mental health services is less austere and authoritarian than that of long-stay institutions. They may take the form of hostels, sheltered accommodation, day centres, workshops or befriending schemes. Often, the size of the organizational setting is reduced and the 'mentally ill' person's family, if any, becomes the main potential source of support. A distinction must be made between care **in** the community and care **by** the community.

At best community mental health care enables people with mental health problems to have their own homes, make their own choices and live their lives with the acceptance of the local community. Unfortunately, it frequently falls short of expectations (O'Brien, 1992; Baker and Intagliata, 1982). Clients may perceive the 'community', in the sense of the social environment in which they live, as their main problem. For example, several respondents in the research described in this chapter complained about the hostel in which they lived and were supposedly 'cared' for. Three people felt that getting out of the hostel would be an adequate solution to their problems!

Community mental health care, as with other forms of community care, implies a reliance on informal support networks. But, for people with mental illness, this network is frequently lacking. In the present research, only three people out of a sample of 29 were married/partnered at the time of the interviews, and two of these identified family pressures as a major problem. It is not adequate to assume that people with family have support, or that providing sheltered accommodation will meet the needs of clients who lack family ties. Community 'care' must respond to individual circumstances and evolving needs.

Who are the mentally ill?

One pragmatic way of delineating the mentally ill is to include all those in receipt of mental health services. In research, it is difficult to avoid this step because it is the easiest way to identify individual cases. However, it cannot be assumed that those in receipt of services have common characteristics. For example, a distinction must be made between those who seek mental health care and those who have it imposed upon them. Neither can it be assumed that people with similar 'symptoms' will define themselves or be defined as mentally ill or be equally likely to seek treatment.

In this chapter, mental illness will be viewed as a social status characterized by the receipt of 'treatment' for 'mental health problems'. Clarke (Chapter 8) and Heyman and Huckle (Chapter 10) made similar moves in connection with dementia and learning difficulties, respectively. They define a 'condition' in terms of a social status, e.g. referral for dementia. The underlying reality is neither affirmed (as with the medical model) or denied (as with labelling theory). Rather, the consequences of this social status are explored with, in the context of the present book, a focus on client perspectives.

From the perspective of a pure medical model, mental illnesses such as schizophrenia and depression can be viewed as caused by biochemical malfunctioning. A social management perspective (Chapter 2) stresses the individual's capacity to play 'normal' roles and so focuses as much on the social environment as on individual impairment and disability.

Many mentally ill people live in circumstances characterized by unstable or non-existent family life and poor socioeconomic circumstances which anyone would find difficult (Franklin *et al.*, 1986). O'Brien (1992) found that only 28% of a sample of recently discharged psychiatric patients had their 'living space' needs met and that only about half of the sample had any work or leisure needs met. Handyside and Heyman (1990) found, in the research discussed in this chapter, that only one out of 29 respondents interviewed was employed at the time of the research.

There has been considerable debate between proponents of social deprivation theories (Faris and Dunham, 1939) who see mental illness as caused by relative poverty and social drift theorists (Myerson, 1941) who believe that mental illness causes social deprivation. Consideration of client perspectives suggests a different kind of approach to this issue. The critical question becomes that of how people with the social status of 'mentally ill' see themselves and explain their own problems, if they think that they have any. Their own perspectives can then be related to those of others, including formal carers.

METHODOLOGY

Background and aims of the research

The research reported here was carried out in part of a large conurbation in the North of England in 1988–9 and was commissioned by a community-based voluntary mental health agency who approached the University of Northumbria. This agency, unlike other community-based mental health services, provided active support to people with mental health problems through relaxation classes, anxiety management and befriending. The service aimed to reduce the likelihood of people being readmitted to hospital by filling the gap between crisis intervention in hospital and medical maintenance in the community.

Its objectives included helping participants to develop practical, domestic and social skills and encouraging them to form supportive links with informal friendship groups and larger clubs and organizations in the community. Intervention was thus directed primarily at changing the implicitly defective ways in which individuals related to the community rather than at psychological symptoms.

The purpose of the research was to evaluate the agency's service and (hopefully) to support an application for further funding. Six months into the study, the agency's management committee decided to terminate the employment of the fieldworker (EH) because they felt that research into clients' perceptions would not provide useful ammunition for grant applications to support the project. There was also considerable tension between staff operating the scheme and members of the management committee. Staff felt that the committee had rather traditional ideas about how to deal with 'mentally ill' people, based on encouraging them to attend a workshop. It just so happened that leading members of the committee had such a scheme running in the same area, in direct competition with the community support scheme!

The research did, however, continue, with EH funding herself through part-time teaching at the University of Northumbria, and a short summary report was sent to the agency on completion.

The main aims of the research were:

- to investigate clients' own perceptions of their problems, their needs and community mental health services;
- to evaluate the effectiveness of the service offered by the voluntary agency (VA) by comparing it with local authority (LA) services in terms of its impact on clients' own assessments of their problems and mental health.

Research design

Quasi-experimental design

The service provided by the voluntary agency was compared with that given by two local authorities in neighbouring districts which had similar social characteristics (a high prevalence of poverty and unemployment) but which did not have the kind of service provided by the VA. Participants in the research were matched, as far as possible, on demographic characteristics and clinical diagnosis (see below).

VA clients were assessed before receiving services and at least three months later. Members of the LA control group were assessed twice over a similar period, with assessment focusing on clients' perceptions of their own problems. The research was thus quasi-experimental and aimed to compare changes in matched groups receiving different 'variants' of a service (Chapter 2) over a three-month period.

LA community mental health care was offered by mental health social workers, community psychiatric nurses and day centres. The priorities seemed to be stabilizing clients' mental health, through administering drugs and reacting to some of their expressed needs. In contrast, the VA offered individual support for each client and actively encouraged the use of anxiety management and relaxation groups run by the scheme.

Hypotheses

The research was designed to test two hypotheses.

1. There will be an improvement in the measured mental health of all groups of respondents between first and second assessment.

2. The measured mental health of the VA group will improve more than that of the control group.

The rationale for the first hypothesis was that clients in both the VA and LA group received treatment and might be expected to improve over time, on average, even without formal care. Greater improvement was expected in the VA group (hypothesis 2) because of the active intervention strategy pursued by the voluntary agency.

The sample

Sample selection and matching

The VA 'experimental' sample was identified fairly randomly by attempting to recruit people who were newly referred to the agency within the time period of the first phase of fieldwork. Sources of referral included clients themselves, social workers, CPNs, family, friends and psychiatrists. GPs and psychologists did not refer anyone to the agency during the research period. Of 12 participants recruited, two dropped out during the research (see below). The experimental group consisted of the remaining 10 new users of the VA service.

LA controls were matched to the VA group with respect to sex, approximate age, marital status and predominant clinical diagnosis. Matching and selection of the control group was done by professional 'gatekeepers' and is discussed below. Because of the scarcity of fully matched controls, matching was not attempted on a one-to-one basis. The aim was to ensure that the VA and LA groups would be similar overall in terms of their predominant problems and social backgrounds.

Originally it was intended to have only one control group (LA1). However, preliminary analysis showed that there was a discrepancy between the VA and LA groups in their place of residence, a variable on which they had not been matched. The majority of the LA1 group lived in hostels and lodgings, whilst most of the VA group lived in their own homes. Respondents themselves considered living circumstances to be a significant influence on their mental health. One VA respondent found the responsibility of home ownership a great strain, whereas two members of the LA group saw having their own home and getting out of the hostel as solutions to their problems.

A second control group (LA2) was therefore selected from another local authority, with matching extended to social circumstances including employment, financial problems and housing as well as assessed clinical condition, age, sex and marital status.

Sampling procedure for control groups and 'gatekeeping'

Matching was achieved by providing local social workers and CPNs with anonymized VA client profiles and asking them to identify a person who was as similar as possible to the VA client and who was likely to be willing to participate in the research. Recruitment of the control groups thus depended on 'gatekeeping' by professionals, without whose help the research would not have been possible.

Three potential problems arose from this method of sample selection. Firstly, gatekeepers might have biased sample selection by unconsciously applying professional ideology, e.g. giving more weight to medical diagnosis than to social circumstances. Secondly, respondents who were approached by 'their' professional might have felt obliged to take part in the study, in case it negatively affected their support, despite repeated and specific assurances to the contrary by the researcher. Thirdly, they might have been more likely to give positive ratings of the professional who introduced them to the study.

Sampling outcomes

It was emphasized that participation in the research was voluntary and that non-participation would not affect individual treatment. The non-participation rate was low. Of the 36 individuals selected for the VA, LA1 and LA2 groups, two could not be contacted and 85% (29) of the remaining 34 potential recruits agreed to take part.

Reasons for refusal included distress at answering questions and fear that association with mental health services would become known to family and friends. One woman was afraid that her husband would find out that she was receiving help from the VA scheme.

A possible reason for the very low refusal rate in this study is that participants, like the elderly residents of sheltered accommodation discussed in Chapter 7, welcomed the opportunity to have somebody to talk to.

Three respondents out of the 29 who completed the first questionnaire were not followed up, two from the VA group and one from LA2. The two VA respondents dropped out due to changes in their personal circumstances, not as a result of the initial interview. The third respondent, from LA2, was excluded by the researcher because he was unable to answer the questions, due to his mental state.

Comparisons of the final samples

The three samples were similar, overall, in age, sex and marital and unemployment status. The only major difference found was, as noted above, the greater number of hostel residents in the LA2 sample. Only one of the 29 respondents was in employment and only three were living with a spouse. The high level of unemployment is significant as respondents frequently mentioned financial problems as a cause of their mental health problems and paid work as a solution.

Methods

A questionnaire, the Circumstances and Health Questionnaire, was developed, combining open and (mostly) closed questions. The questionnaire was designed to reliably assess clients' biographical details, perceptions of their problems, use of and satisfaction with services and general mental health.

Ratings of satisfaction with services were based on part of the Consumer Satisfaction Schedule (Catalan *et al.*, 1980). Mental health was assessed through 72 questions about psychological states (e.g. anxiety, depression, irritability) derived from three reputable rating scales. These were the State-Trait Anxiety Inventory (Spielberger, Gorusch and Lushene, 1970), the Wakefield Self-Assessment Depression Inventory (Snaith, Ahmed and Metha, 1971) and part of the 30-item General Health Questionnaire (Goldberg and Hillier, 1979).

Although derived from three different sources, total scores were highly consistent. The split-half reliability of the 72-item scale (with Spearman-Brown correction) was 0.91 at Time One, and 0.95 at Time Two. (This statistic indicates that individuals' total score on odd-numbered questions, i.e. the first, third, fifth, etc., predicted, almost perfectly, their scores on even numbered items. Perfect reliability would be indicated by a correlation of 1.0.) It was therefore meaningful to derive a single score from the full 72 questions, since they appeared to be measuring a consistent property of individuals.

Test–retest reliability was 0.79, demonstrating that individuals more or less maintained their relative mental health 'scores' over the three-month period of the research even though, as will be shown below, average scores improved. (Test–retest reliability was assessed by correlating individuals' scores at Times One and Two. One problem with such measures is that they do not allow real relative changes, e.g. one person improving more than another, to be differentiated from measurement inaccuracies.)

Validity was assessed by 'triangulating' questionnaire results with qualitative assessments of respondents' own self-reported problems. Good agreement was obtained, as will be shown in the Results section.

It was originally intended that the questionnaire be self-completing, but piloting showed that some respondents were illiterate or felt very uncomfortable about writing. In the main study, the questionnaire was used as a structured interview schedule with the interviewer (EH) recording replies verbatim.

One advantage of adopting a structured interview format was that it was possible to record qualitative detail as well as specific responses to closed questions. For example, when asked what they thought were their main problems, respondents tended to answer in great detail and then ask which bits they should write down! The researcher was able to record the detail as well as the final answer. Tape-recording might have assisted the process of recording detail, but might have inhibited respondents or made it more difficult for them to accept that their identity and responses would remain confidential.

RESULTS

Introduction

Results from the two LA groups were similar and were combined for analysis. Quantitative comparisons were made between the VA and combined LA groups for mental health scores, frequency of contact with community health care professionals and evaluations of these contacts. Changes in respondents' qualitative accounts of their problems were then related to changes in mental health scores.

Comparisons of mental health scores

Comparisons of mental health scores at Times One and Two, for the entire sample and for the VA and LA groups separately are displayed in Table 11.1.

Table 11.1 Changes in mean self-ratings of mental health in the voluntary agency and combined local authority groups ($n = 26$)

Comparison	Time One	Time Two	Change Time One–Time Two
Full sample ($n = 26$)	2.70$_a$	3.00$_a$	+ 0.30
Voluntary agency group ($n = 10$)	2.66	2.90	+ 0.24$_b$
Local authority group ($n = 16$)	2.73	3.05	+ 0.32$_b$

Higher scores indicate better self-rated mental health
Positive change scores indicate improvements in self-reported mental health
a Change between Time One and Time Two for the whole sample statistically significant at < 0.005 level (related t test–$t = 2.7$).
b Changes in VA self-reported mental health scores not significantly different from changes in LA group (one-way analysis of variance – $F_{1,24} = 0.12$)

Quantitative analysis supported hypothesis 1, that the average self-reported mental health of both groups would improve significantly over time.

The second hypothesis was that positive changes in self-reported mental health would be greater for the VA than the LA group. However, the results shown in Table 11.1 do not support this hypothesis, as the amount of positive change was slightly, but insignificantly, greater in the LA group.

Frequency of contact with professionals

One partial indicator of the quality of person-centred services is the frequency with which professionals make contact with their clients (Bond, 1990). Respondents had most frequent contact with CPNs, followed by social workers, and had least contact with psychiatrists and psychologists. Contacts were significantly less frequent at Time Two than Time One. This reduction in contact may have resulted from improvements in overall mental health of the sample over time, as discussed above. Alternatively, it might reflect a gradual loss of attention by community mental health services.

The LA group had, on average, had contact with a mental health professional significantly more recently (mean time = 0.7 months, n = 19) than the VA group (mean time = 1.6 months, n = 10) at Time One (related t = 2.58 with 25 df, p >0.05). At Time Two, members of the LA group still had more recent contacts than the VA group, but the difference was not statistically significant. One explanation of the Time One difference is that individuals sought or were referred to the VA service because they were receiving less formal care.

Ratings of professionals

Respondents were asked to rate the professionals with whom they had contact on six five-point scales. An average score of 1, the most favourable score possible, would have indicated that the professional was rated as very easy to talk to, interested in the client, helpful, understanding and good at his/her job. Average ratings of all these professionals were, on balance, favourable.

There were some very positive comments about health professionals.

He [psychiatrist] made a path for me to follow. Otherwise I would probably still be going round in circles. (Respondent AC)

Some respondents had a disturbing degree of faith in modern medicine.

He's a doctor, so he has to understand. (Respondent WR)

Reservations and criticisms were expressed, however. One patient, who rated her CPN highly, felt that there were limits to the extent to which a professional who had not experienced mental distress could help someone who had.

There's a limit to how good you [CPN] can be if you haven't been through it yourself. (Respondent RC)

Her words evoke the quotation from Strauss and Corbin (1988), discussed in Chapter 1, suggesting that people with chronic health problems and professional carers inhabit separate worlds.

Problems sometimes arose because the patient did not accept the diagnosis and, implicitly, the medical model.

> When the doctor told me I was schizophrenic, I didn't believe him. I thought I was just seeing visions because of what had happened [mother dying and girlfriend leaving].... I would like to have visions now. I would like to prove that I am psychic rather than schizophrenic. (Respondent SM)

A few patients felt that they had suffered iatrogenic disease, probably with good reason in the light of current views about tranquillizer addiction.

> In the past I was put on tranquillizers for 'nerves', and then I suddenly stopped. I didn't realize that I would feel like living hell.... If I had more literature, then I would have realized that it was all withdrawal. (Respondent BR)

Overall, respondents rated their contact with CPNs and social workers more favourably than those with psychiatrists and psychologists. CPNs and social workers were also seen most frequently. However, among the 19 respondents who were seeing a CPN, this professional was rated less favourably by the VA group (mean = 2.4, n = 7 at Time One) than by the LA group (mean = 1.2, n = 12 at Time One). One-way analysis of variance showed that this difference was statistically significant ($F_{1,17}$ = 16.99, p = >0.001). Similar differences were found for Time Two ratings.

No significant differences were found in VA and LA evaluations of the other professionals. Because the numbers were so small, the difference in rating of the CPN must be interpreted with caution, but three related explanations can be suggested. Firstly, clients who were disenchanted with the CPN service might have turned to the VA as an alternative source of support. Secondly, CPNs, who frequently referred their clients to the VA, might have passed on the most 'difficult' cases, e.g. the non-compliant. Thirdly, the feeling of being passed on to another service might have made VA respondents feel less favourable towards CPNs.

Predominant mental health problems

Each respondent was asked, through an open-ended question, what they perceived to be their main problems. Not surprisingly, the types of problem reported varied widely (see Table 11.2 for examples). Some individuals gave mainly psychological accounts of their problems (e.g. anxiety, depression) while others defined their problems situationally (e.g. lack of a job, poor living conditions) or gave mixed descriptions. As discussed below, improvements in mental health scores were associated with a shift towards more social situational explanations of problems.

The clinical diagnoses that respondents mentioned included depression, schizophrenia, anxiety, nerves, panic attacks, fear and hallucinations. In some cases, these appeared to be no more than labels which professionals had given to the respondent and which meant very little to them. One man, described by both his social worker and CPN as a chronic schizophrenic, for which he was receiving medication, seemed unaware of this diagnosis and perceived his problems to be situational, e.g. not working, getting bored and taking tablets.

> If I could get a job I'd feel better. (Respondent GD)

Respondents gave far more emphasis to their current situation than clinical symptoms in explaining their problems, e.g. lack of money, not getting out, not having a job, boredom, living in a 'rough' area or a hostel, taking pills, or not sleeping.

However, the importance of the social status of having a medically defined illness was not lost on some people. The respondent quoted below appeared to have accepted medication, despite concern about its effects, in order to qualify for sickness benefit.

> That's another thing, you have no rights because they stop your benefit. You have your benefit because you are sick, but if you refuse treatment you shouldn't have the benefit. The treatment just numbs you. (Respondent CP)

As well as seeing iatrogenic effects of their medical treatment, some respondents had a strong sense of the socially stigmatizing effects of the 'mental illness' label.

> I don't want to meet people because I feel they look at you strangely because of the illness, but you can't just tell them because of the stigma. (Respondent PR)

Diagnostic categories applied to the participants in this study appeared to describe a large variety of misunderstood and strange behaviours. For example, there were wide variations in the types and severity of so called 'schizophrenic symptoms'. But there was only one instance when the respondent was so detached from reality at the time of the interview that it seemed impossible to communicate with him.

Questionnaire changes and qualitative assessment

Participants' self-reported problems were compared, case by case, with the quantitative measure of mental health. Summaries for the five cases showing the most positive and most negative change scores are presented in Table 11.2.

Table 11.2 Self-reported problems and mental health change scores

	Time One	*Time Two*
Most favourable changes in mental health scores		
Male; 47 VA; +1.07 Divorced Unemployed	Schizophrenia Anxiety Suicidal thoughts	Worry over rent
Male; 43 LA; +0.99 Single Unemployed	Schizophrenia Physical sensations No money Not sleeping	No money No social life Not going anywhere
Male; 37 LA; +0.94 Single Unemployed	Visions/hallucinations Mood swings	No problems
Female; 45 LA; +0.94 Married Employed	Anxiety; nerves Dizziness; headaches Not sleeping Breathing problems	Anxious about job Dizziness Blood pressure Changing GPs
Male; 58 VA; +0.90 Single Unemployed	No money Not getting out Getting lost	No place of own
Least favourable changes in mental health scores		
Female; 68 LA; –0.75 Widowed Retired	Anxiety; panic attacks Upset/screaming Agoraphobia Unhappy	Feeling a nuisance Panic attacks Getting in a state Agoraphobia; lethargy
Female; 55 VA; –0.68 Widowed Unemployed	Nervous breakdown Nerves/tension Being homeless Heart attack	Worried; frightened Being on own Living in hostel Not making decision
Female; 28 VA; –0.54 Single Unemployed	Agoraphobia; anxiety Depression Coping with mother Cramp in legs	Agoraphobia Depression
Female; 27 VA; –0.35 Single Unemployed	Feeling cut off Afraid to go out Panic; depression Anger with self	Panic Anxiety Depression
Male; 40 VA; –0.34 Single Unemployed	Nervous; depression Fear Horrible feelings Tense with others	Nervous; depression Mixing socially Fitting in

Several trends can be seen in Table 11.2. Firstly, there was a marked reduction in the range of problems reported by the positive change group at Time Two and little evidence of such a shift in the negative change group.

Secondly, those problems which the positive change group did report at Time Two were much more likely to be socially referenced (e.g. isolation, job, living circumstances) rather than psychologically referenced (e.g. anxiety, depression) than at Time One. Such a shift in client perspectives on their problems was not evident in the negative change group.

Thirdly, although men did not differ significantly from women overall in their mental health scores, it is noticeable that four of the clients who changed most positively were men while four of those who changed most negatively were women. The woman who registered a high positive change in mental health was unusual in that she was married, employed and a home owner. This finding suggests that single unemployed women may find it more difficult to recover their mental health in our society.

DISCUSSION

Quantitative change in mental health

The apparent improvement in measured mental health by both client groups might not reflect real changes in mental health. It may have been, in whole or in part, a result of testing effects, i.e. respondents reacting differently to questions which they were answering for a second time (Cook and Campbell, 1979).

However, the detailed case notes suggest that real changes were taking place and that these corresponded on the whole to changes indicated by the questionnaire. Individuals who registered improvements on the questionnaire reported fewer problems at Time Two. The problems that they did mention were more likely to have a social rather than a psychological referent. Such changes were not evident in individuals whose mental health, as measured by the questionnaire, had become worse.

It cannot be assumed that positive changes were caused by professional interventions, since there is no way of knowing if clients would have improved even in the absence of such intervention.

It was predicted that the more active and participatory support offered by the VA would result in greater improvements in mental health than the support offered by the LA services. This hypothesis was not supported. Although not encouraging, this finding does not demonstrate that the VA services were not in any way beneficial. It is possible that the mental health measure and the qualitative assessment in the interview failed to detect changes which had occurred, that the limited three-month time-frame of the study excluded changes happening in the longer term, that changes would have been detected with larger samples or that the specific form of the VA intervention was not effective.

Why the VA intervention might have been ineffective

If the failure of the VA scheme was genuine, rather than a methodological artefact, two explanations for its lack of success can be given.

Differences between the VA and LA group

Firstly, although great efforts were made to match individuals in the VA and LA groups, the quasi-experimental nature of the design meant that the one variable on which they could not be matched was the decision of VA clients to refer themselves, or be referred to, the voluntary agency. The VA group were receiving significantly less frequent contacts with formal services at the time when they enrolled with the VA and were significantly more critical of CPNs, the most frequently contacted professionals. Such selection effects could only have been eliminated in a fully randomized experiment, which the organizations involved in the study would not have allowed and which would have raised ethical and methodological problems.

Members of the VA group might have joined the voluntary agency because they were dissatisfied with the formal services they were receiving. It is possible that the VA was supporting people whose needs were not being met by statutory services and that this benefit was not detected because of the quasi-experimental design of the study.

A social situational explanation

Alternatively, the apparent failure of the VA scheme may reflect the intrinsic ineffectiveness of interventions aimed at the individual. Attempts to improve the mental health of people living in the community through personal support may be doomed to failure, because the main 'cause' of 'mental' problems is located not primarily in individuals' minds, but in their bleak social circumstances. Long-term unemployment, lack of a spouse or partner and inadequate housing were almost universal among sample members.

There is considerable research evidence for a relationship between adverse social circumstances and poor mental health, e.g. unemployment (Furnham, 1983; Roy, 1987; Westcott, 1987) and living alone (Nieminen, 1986; Hanson and Ostergren, 1987).

Although the direction of causality cannot be determined in these studies it is likely that there is a positive feedback loop between adverse social circumstances and poor mental health. Adverse social circumstances may lead to mental health problems, while mental health problems may result in a deterioration of social circumstances through, for example, inability to get a job.

Qualitative and quantitative assessments of mental health

Perhaps the most interesting finding of the study was the relationship between the quantitative measure of change in self-reported mental health, derived from closed questions, and the qualitative measure, based on answers to open-ended questions. Respondents whose measured mental health improved over the three months of the study showed signs not only of a reduction in the number of problems that they mentioned, as might be expected, but also a qualitative shift in the kinds of problem that concerned them. Improvement was associated with a marked shift from psychological to social situational referents for their problems.

For some clients, at least, whose underlying problems are associated with their social situation, poor mental health may simply mean that their psychological responses to social deprivation (e.g. anxiety, depression, confusion) become their central problems. This psychological response may temporarily or permanently 'blot out' clients' awareness of the social circumstances that gave rise to poor mental health, while partially improved mental health leads to rediscovery of the underlying social problem. 'Treatment' of problems such as unemployment, poverty and social isolation cannot be achieved through psychological interventions or medication because they have a wider societal dimension, and require political change involving society as a whole.

CHAPTER 12

The needs of people with HIV, their informal carers and service providers

Elizabeth Handyside

INTRODUCTION

This chapter discusses a study of the needs of people infected with HIV and the services provided for them. The research was carried out between 1992 and 1994 in North Yorkshire, an area of low HIV prevalence, and was commissioned by the new North Yorkshire Health Authority (NYHA). Three factors were instrumental in the decision for the research to proceed: the purchaser/provider split, the creation of a new health authority and rumours of dissatisfaction with local HIV services among key workers and users.

Following the purchaser/provider split initiated by the NHS and Community Care Act 1990, purchasers were required to draw up contracts with the most suitable people to provide services to meet the needs of local service users. For contracting to be successful, purchasers have to assess local need and demand for health care and appraise service options. The NYHA arose from the amalgamation of five Yorkshire health authorities and became responsible for joint purchasing.

In the year preceding these changes, several HIV workers had heard rumours of dissatisfaction with local services. Also, local people with HIV were opting to use services in neighbouring health authorities and elsewhere. A need was identified to make an 'objective' and comprehensive assessment of the local HIV services, in order to provide a basis for improvements.

The language of HIV and AIDS frequently reflects the prejudice and discrimination that surrounds people with the illness. Throughout the chapter, I shall use the phrase **HIV-positives** (HPs) as a neutral term (see Chapter 1) to describe people with HIV, HIV-related illness or AIDS. The partners, family and friends who provide care for HPs will be called **informal carers**. I will use the term **service provider** to describe the health, social or voluntary sector workers who provide care for people affected by HIV.

I will first highlight the key issues in the literature relating to community care for people with HIV. I will then outline the research methodology, drawing attention to problems of confidentiality and gatekeeping, before discussing the research findings.

The prevalence of HIV and AIDS in North Yorkshire

Accurate figures on the incidence and prevalence of HIV and AIDS are not available nationally or locally and the distinction between HIV-related illness and AIDS is imprecise. Between 1987 and 1993, about 30 AIDS and 35 HIV cases have been identified in North Yorkshire. Services, therefore, have to meet the needs of a small number of people in an area of low prevalence. However, my research suggests that these figures may be underestimates.

HIV and community care

The advent of HIV has challenged existing community and hospital, statutory and voluntary, health and social systems of care. Many people affected by HIV are unwilling to accept inappropriate or inadequate services. The chronic nature of HIV and early detection of the virus, coupled with the relative youth of many affected people, have provided a unique opportunity for users to plan and develop their own services. As a result, the HIV/AIDS 'community' has become active in restructuring existing services and developing new voluntary services to better meet their needs.

It is about 20 years since the first cases became known. In that time the 'fight against AIDS' has gathered immense support, but the struggle for comprehensive, sensitive and expert care continues. The needs of people with HIV/AIDS can best be met through community based services (Cunningham, 1989; McEwan, 1989; McCann and Wadsworth, 1992). But problems in delivering such care stem from the diverse clinical demands of HIV-related illnesses, and from the stigma associated with HIV and AIDS (Layzell and McCarthy, 1992).

Community-based HIV services

Both service users and service providers want community-based HIV services. People with HIV may argue that community services are more accessible and flexible than hospital services and that the control and coordination of services remains with the 'patient'. Others may prefer the demedicalization and relative comfort of home care, or argue that home care provides a sense of normalization, particularly when a partner or parent plays an important role in caring. Service providers and planners perceive advantages of community care for people with HIV in terms of logistics (e.g. hospital bed space) and cost.

McEwan (1992) states that the aim of community care for people with HIV should be: 'to enable an individual to remain in his own home wherever possible rather than being cared for permanently in a hospital or residential home' (p. 23). McEwan further suggests that there should be a range of community services to match the range and complexity of medical and social needs of people with HIV.

McCann (1990) argues that, in reality, care in the community is care by the community, namely informal carers, volunteers and other community members.

The organization of community-based services

Layzell and McCarthy (1992) suggest three important aspects of the success of community care for people with HIV: the need for collaborative work, case management and the debate about the merits of specialist and generic services.

Collaboration

Originally HIV/AIDS was seen as a primarily medical problem. As the chronic nature of the illness became apparent, additional financial and social problems were identified. These required 'packages' of care involving collaboration between health, social and voluntary services. There are some outstanding examples of collaborative community care, including the London Lighthouse (Thompson, 1989) and the Landmark (Grimshaw, 1989). Layzell and McCarthy (1992) suggest that collaboration depends upon individual commitment and relationships rather than central direction. Collaboration may therefore be somewhat fragile, given the differences in ideology and group identification that exist in the caring professions.

Case management

Case management is a possible solution to the problem of coordinating services. It has been described as 'the cornerstone of community care' (Shepherd, 1990), in that it increases access to services and enhances patient and carer satisfaction.

A case worker may operate as an 'agency broker' by coordinating services and clients, or as a more therapeutic 'key worker'. The literature on the psychosocial needs of HIV service users suggests that the latter is more appropriate (Salisbury, 1986; Reidy, Taggart and Asselin, 1991). But the success of this approach rather riskily depends on the development of a good relationship between key worker and client. As Layzell and McCarthy (1992) note, there is considerable potential for interprofessional rivalry.

Benjamin (1989) researched HIV/AIDS case management in the USA. He suggested that case management reduces unmet need and improves use of non-institutional services, but has little effect on client health and use of institutional services. Its cost, in the USA at least, is greater than that of alternative approaches to HIV care.

In the UK there are examples of specialist HIV/AIDS home support teams whose role includes coordination between hospital and community care, but is not reliant on one key worker. McCann (1991) found that clients rated such teams favourably, not only in terms of their coordinating and facilitating role but also in terms of support, advice and counselling. For some respondents, just the existence of the team was reassuring.

Special home support teams may be the key to community care for people with HIV and AIDS. But, where prevalence is low and doesn't warrant such a specialist team, the responsibility for HIV care in the community tends to fall on GPs and district nurses. This can mean a fragmented and inexpert service, as GPs are not HIV specialists, and can increase pressure on family, volunteers and non-community practitioners to fill the gaps (McCann, 1991).

Roderick, Victor and Beardhow (1990) found that a large proportion of (London-based) GPs wanted to be involved with HIV/AIDS patients. But these GPs felt that before taking such patients they needed information, education and counselling skills. The majority only wanted to be involved in shared care of people with HIV/AIDS. There was a reluctance to deal with intravenous drug users and homosexuals. These GPs appeared willing to take on only a relatively small proportion of HIV patients.

Specialist versus generic services

If existing community-based services are unable to provide the type of flexible, sensitive and expert service that people with HIV/AIDS demand, then perhaps the provision of specialist HIV services should be considered. Service users argue that specialist HIV services, employing designated HIV workers, can reduce stigma by encouraging acceptance and expertise (King, 1989). However, separate HIV services may increase stigma by creating segregated services and 'hamper the long-term objective of normalization of AIDS' (Cunningham, 1989).

In practice, some in-patient services have unwittingly developed a reputation as specialist providers, as a growing number of people with HIV/AIDS present with similar clinical problems such as chest complaints and specific cancers. This increased experience of HIV may lead service providers to develop expertise and to be increasingly sought by service users.

The variable prevalence of HIV may bias the decision between specialist or generic services. Typically, services in areas like North Yorkshire, where HIV prevalence is low, have evolved reactively and almost haphazardly around existing service providers (Cunningham, 1989). Such service providers may be less willing to oblige if their HIV caseload has increased, their non-HIV patient caseload has not decreased and they have been dubbed the local 'AIDS expert'.

Cunningham (1989) argues that the absorption of HIV patients into generic services is cost-effective and avoids unnecessary duplication of community services such as district nursing. There is a danger that providing specialist HIV services will exclude the use of existing expertise, e.g. provision of terminal care by Macmillan nurses. But it is increasingly more difficult for generic services to meet the often time-consuming and intensive care needs of people with HIV. There is also the problem of defining the cut-off point, in terms of prevalence within an area, at which specialist services may be justified.

METHODOLOGY

Introduction

The research aimed to build a picture of current local HIV services through interviews with key providers, HPs living or using services in North Yorkshire and current or bereaved informal carers.

Practical constraints meant that interviews did not take place concurrently. The three groups of respondents were interviewed consecutively over a one-year period. The purpose of this design was to be able to 'triangulate' the data from the three sets of interviews and elicit common and opposing viewpoints on which to base recommendations for changes in services.

The research objectives were to investigate:

- the needs of HPs and their informal carers;
- the perceived satisfaction of users with current service provision and possible areas of change;
- the needs and skills of service providers;
- patterns of service use in North Yorkshire and outside;
- organization of services within and between districts.

Due to rapid changes resulting from contracting, some services had changed in the time-span between interviewing service providers, HPs and informal carers. However, respondents tended to have created an impression of services based on their experiences over a long period, unaffected by current change.

The research was overseen by a multiagency research committee. I came to see this group as a means of diffusing responsibility and legit-imizing my decisions. Piloting and sampling were facilitated by assur-ances that all interview schedules had been approved by the committee.

The sample

Service providers

The first stage of the investigation was to meet the five HIV prevention coordinators in North Yorkshire, and to gather outline data about key services in each locality. This process resulted in a target population of about 50 'key' service providers, reduced to 36 with help from the research committee.

Recruiting letters were sent to these 36 HIV service providers. It proved impossible to arrange interviews with three of the sample, due to the pressure of their work, and three refused to participate on the grounds that they would have nothing to contribute. Service providers were drawn from statutory health and social services and voluntary and non-statutory AIDS and drugs agencies. The distribution of the service provider sample was skewed towards localities within North Yorkshire of greater HIV prevalence, reflecting the greater variety of services provided in these areas.

HIV-positives

HPs and informal carers were sampled through service provider contacts. I anticipated that the sample of HPs would snowball through the network of local people with HIV, and that the informal carer sample would come from contacts with HPs. In fact, the network was less apparent than I had anticipated. None of the HPs was able or willing to recruit others.

Contacting people with HIV is a difficult process. Because of the emphasis on confidentiality, the sample must be self-selecting. In this research, contacting HPs was further complicated by gatekeeping.

Of the 30 service providers interviewed, only 12 (40%) said that they were currently in touch with HPs. The number of contacts ranged from one to 10. Each was asked (verbally and by letter) if they would pass on information to 'their' HPs. A further eight service providers or HIV agen-cies thought to be in contact with HPs in North Yorkshire were asked to help with recruitment. Potential contacts were asked to hand out written information about participation in the research, and how to contact me. Assurances of confidentiality were given at every stage.

This process yielded just six interviews with HP service users over a 12-month period. The sample was (unavoidably) biased, since four of the six

HPs interviewed were contacted through a single service provider. Service provider 'gatekeepers' may have been reluctant to provide contacts for several reasons. They may not have been convinced about the practical value of the research or may not have understood the importance of needs assessment in contracting. They may have felt defensive because their roles were being evaluated or concerned that relationships with new clients might be jeopardized. In contrast, for the pilot study, I was easily able to recruit five HPs from a neighbouring area with a higher prevalence of HIV, through a well-used drop-in centre.

All six respondents were male. Their ages ranged between 22 and 50 years (mean = 35.3 years). Five described themselves as 'gay' and one was a heterosexual haemophiliac. Two lived with a partner/spouse whom they identified as their carer. Four were single (one bereaved). Three of these four lived alone and had no informal carer. The other lived with an elderly relative who did not know of his positive status and was not a carer.

Three of the sample lived in a rural and three in an urban area. Only two were in full-time paid employment, the others having left work since their diagnosis, although one person did part-time voluntary work. At the time of the interview, the average length of unemployment was 27 months (range 5 months–5 years), and five HPs were claiming benefits.

At the time of the interview, the average length of time since diagnosis was 5 years 6 months (range 6 months–10 years). Only one HP had voluntarily presented himself for a test. Two were tested during routine screening. The other three had had an HIV test at the suggestion of their doctor. Three described themselves as symptomatic, one as asymptomatic, and the other two were intermediate. All were on medications, including prophylactics, antibiotics, pain killers and tranquillizers.

Informal carers

A separate sample of five informal carers, three female, two male, were recruited. Two were bereaved and three currently living with and caring for an HP.

The average carer age was 49.6 years (range 36–58 years). Three had (non-HIV) health problems and two had left work as a result. Two other sample members left work to look after their HP partner/relative. Only one person was employed, while caring for her son.

Two carers were mothers of the HP, two were partners and one was a brother-in-law who looked after the HP while he was very ill, over a period of two weeks.

All carers except the latter had cared for the HP over a longish period, averaging 3.7 years (range 1.3–9.5 years). The intensity of caring varied, depending on the degree of illness of the HP.

Methods

Face-to-face semi-structured interviews were carried out with all respondents from each of the three samples. The interview schedules were specifically designed to relate to one another so that comparisons between the views of HPs, service providers and informal carers could be made. All interview schedules were passed by the local ethics committees and piloted in neighbouring areas prior to use in the main study. Interviews were mainly qualitative.

On average, interviews with HPs lasted 2 hours and those with informal carers 1.7 hours. All interviews were carried out by the researcher, in private, at a venue chosen by the respondent. Most HPs and informal carers were interviewed at home, but two HPs wished to be interviewed at the office of a familiar service provider. Prior to interview, all respondents were assured that their identity and responses would remain confidential to the interviewer. All HPs and informal carers gave written consent.

Notes were taken during the interview and written up afterwards with comments. Interviews were not taped, as it was felt that this might lead to further insecurity regarding confidentiality.

The data were analysed using a grounded theory approach (Strauss and Corbin, 1990). Important recurrent themes quickly emerged from the service provider data. These were used to 'sensitize' the data collected in HP and informal carer interviews. Pertinent themes which occurred frequently, sometimes because of references in the interview schedule, were reinvestigated by closer examination of the data, and comparisons between and within the three samples.

RESULTS

Introduction

The results will be reported in stages roughly corresponding to the likely sequence of events in the service-use career of an HP. I will start by discussing levels of knowledge about HIV and HIV services and highlight the difference between theoretical and practical knowledge. I will show how lack of knowledge can result in haphazard service use and indicate the importance of first impressions for later service use. The desire for independence and self-help amongst HPs will be related to finance and the effects of chronic illness. Lastly, I will discuss symptomatic HPs' concern for continuity and their desire for specific HIV services.

Knowledge about HIV

HPs and informal carers, generally, had known little about HIV before it became a personal issue for them. Four of the 11 HPs and informal carers had nursed an HIV-positive partner or had close HP friends. One informal carer, not HIV-positive, was currently looking after his third HP partner. Amongst the inexperienced, the main sources of information (and misinformation) were library books and the media, particularly TV. Several carers made the distinction between theoretical knowledge and practical experience.

> We'd read a lot about HIV, not that that helps you confront it, but it removes the fear. (IC2)

The fulfilment of informal carers' information needs may be related to the HP's degree of acceptance of his/her positive status. One informal carer was acutely aware of her own lack of knowledge even though her husband had been diagnosed for almost 10 years. Her ignorance may have been associated with her husband's denial of his positive status and her consequent lack of access to sources of information. She was particularly concerned about the progression of his illness and would liked to have been in touch with other carers for support.

Her husband, quoted below, was unaware of her desire for information and support.

> I'd rather not know if I'm going to die.... I don't know of anyone else (with HIV). I'm not interested. I want to forget it. They used to have a group [at the clinic], but it's not my cup of tea, or my wife's. (HP5)

Informal carers may be allied to service providers in their caring role, but they are also service users with individual needs. Meeting conflicting needs for information poses 'wicked problems' for service providers.

The distinction between HIV theory and practical experience has implications for the training of service providers. HPs in this and other studies (Beedham and Wilson-Barnett, 1991) have called for training which focuses more on what it means to have HIV. However, service providers in this study were more concerned with the need for clinical updates. They did not express a need for training which would enhance their awareness of 'being' HIV-positive.

> Most people involved have a sound basic knowledge. We need updates on medical progression and the social scene. (Social Worker 1)

The benefit of learning through sharing experiences, rather than through training, was acknowledged by some service providers.

> I've learnt more about the disease, and people's ability to cope with horrifying situations and their incredible strength. This sort of expe-

rience influences the way you treat people in the future, more so than education. (GP1)

Service users tended to assume that practitioners at the top of the medical hierarchy had superior knowledge. However, the five consultants interviewed did not share this view.

I train myself through journals and books. I have picked up counselling skills by talking to people. This is not adequate, but there is no time allowed for courses. (Consultant J)

Unofficially, consultants obtained information from their colleagues. One admitted that he had learnt about HIV from a nurse colleague with greater experience, and another through his patients.

HIV people are very well informed, and I can learn from them. (Consultant D)

Initial experiences of HIV services

For many HPs, their first experience of HIV services is receiving a test with a positive result. All HPs described this as a significant and potentially traumatic event. The processes leading to diagnosis and the attitudes of service providers often made matters worse. A common complaint among HPs was the length of time that they had to wait between testing and results.

One HP was certain that he was 'in the clear' because over two months elapsed between him being tested and receiving his result. His reaction was to be resigned to the inadequacy of the health service.

Like with everything else in the NHS, you just accept it. You just get very cynical. (HP4)

Another HP had to wait four months for his test result, but was spared from mental anguish at the time because he was unaware that he had been tested. However, once he did discover his status, he had to deal not only with the shock but also with the retrospective knowledge that, unaware that he might be HIV-positive, he had made some disastrous business decisions.

I was very, very angry. I felt bitter and cheated especially as I had made decisions that I wouldn't, had I known that I had been tested. (HP3)

Both of these HPs were tested some years ago. Although the standards of testing procedures have improved, a recently tested respondent still had to wait three weeks for his results. The analysis of blood for HIV takes less than one hour.

Post-test counselling was commonly thought to be inadequate, focusing on practical advice and restrictive behaviour, rarely on emotional issues. One HP described his recent post-test experience.

> He explained what HIV was, but I got no sympathy, no information, no telephone numbers or leaflets, and was told of no-one who could help me. He said I could go back, and I did once, but he just repeated everything. There was no counselling. (HP6)

However, the service provider described above felt that the service he offered adequately met clients' needs.

> I provide ongoing counselling and support if someone is positive.... The positive people come back formally every three months for a full physical evaluation, a T cell count and a talk through their anxieties. There is an offer to come in at other times for a chat. People are told about other options that are available for help.... People are happy to come back ... so we must be fulfilling a need. (Genito-urinary Nurse 1)

The above quotations document a substantial gap between provider and user perspectives. The HP's perspective might have been coloured by the bad news of his positive test result (Bond, 1990).

First impressions count

Service users' first impressions are likely to influence their decisions about later use. HPs who were unhappy with testing or other services tended to travel elsewhere for follow-up. One HP and his positive partner tried HIV services in four different localities in 18 months because they were unhappy about the way they were treated. Others suggested that they weren't prepared to use certain services because of their poor reputation.

> I would be very wary of using the volunteer services. From what I've heard [from other HPs] I wouldn't be confident that given volunteers would maintain confidentiality. (HP5)

A recently tested respondent judged that carer attitude and practical experience were inadequate.

> I felt as though they wanted to brush it under the carpet. It needs to be out more. I felt like any other person, not special. If they want people to go there [local genito-urinary service] they should get proper HIV people. (HP6)

This respondent chose to use follow-up services elsewhere, and found them to be accepting, efficient and helpful. He liked the simplicity of all his needs being met by a central resource.

When I go there, I only see one person. I don't want to get passed around. (HP6)

Once HPs had established an acceptable system of care and personal relationships with service providers, they were reluctant to change. One HP explained that he didn't want to move to local services, despite the convenience, because it would mean developing new relationships with service providers. Since service users are likely to maintain patterns of care once they are established, service providers need to make the initial contact as supportive as possible.

Choosing HIV services

The services that HPs reported using included specialist nurses, GPs, consultants, genito-urinary departments, specialist counsellors, workers for voluntary HIV agencies, social workers and community psychiatric nurses. The mean number of services used was 4.5 (range 3–7). This system of community care can be compared with those for people with dementia (Chapter 8) and the mentally ill (Chapter 11) in that a wide range of agencies were involved and individual patterns of referral varied. It will be argued below that the resulting overall system of care was haphazard and uncoordinated.

In terms of the location of services, three HPs used North Yorkshire services, and three travelled to larger centres (one to Leeds and two to London).

How do HPs decide where to go for services, and what choices do they have? Real choice is limited by lack of knowledge of what is available. Some HPs felt that they were not given sufficient information about other services by the initial contact. One respondent described how, following his test at the genito-urinary clinic, he was told of no-one, other than the genito-urinary staff, who might offer help or support.

Initially there was no-one until I asked about benefits, and was referred to the social worker, and then she put me in touch with [main community HIV worker]. (HP5)

GPs and other non-HIV-specific community workers were unlikely to have comprehensive knowledge of HIV services.

Often a patient is passive and agreeable to whatever the doctor suggests.... This is to do with the patient's lack of knowledge. All choices could be offered if I have the knowledge, but I don't have this. (GP1)

Failure to inform HPs about other available services might have resulted from service providers' lack of knowledge, possessiveness towards clients or narrow definitions of their roles.

HPs indicated that they were either left to discover services for themselves or were passed from one professional to another. There was little indication that use of HIV services was governed by informed choice. When asked about important support, carers and HPs emphasized the need for 'signposting' through the system.

We need knowledge of what is available. Once you know, it's up to you to take advantage. (IC2)

Several informal carers described avoidable struggles resulting from lack of recommendation by service providers.

As good a GP as he was, he never suggested going to anyone else, perhaps because he didn't know of anyone. We had to find out about the consultant for ourselves.... I'd have liked to have known what was available sooner. I struggled on before I realized what was possible. (IC3)

Confidentiality

HPs perceived a close interrelationship between confidentiality maintenance and the quality of a service.

If a service is good, confidentiality will follow. (HP1)

Many service providers were aware of the importance of confidentiality but admitted that occasional 'innocent' or 'unintentional' breaches occurred. A district nurse explained, for example, that working on a rota and discussing case notes with colleagues made it more likely that a patient's identity would be revealed.

No matter how unintentional, any risk to confidentiality was treated seriously by HPs. Even isolated breaches could permanently damage a service's reputation. For example, a local voluntary organization had developed a poor reputation for confidentiality due to the actions of one of its volunteers who had left five years previously. Five of six HPs in the sample mentioned this as a reason for not wanting to use the service.

Independence of HIV-positive people

Another reason for choosing not to use a service was wanting to remain independent. This may be important to HPs, but can increase strain on informal carers. One informal carer described how she rejected the offer of nightsitting services, despite needing a good night's sleep, because she respected her HIV-positive son's wish to be 'independent'. Again the divergence of needs between HPs and informal carers is apparent.

The ability of HPs to remain relatively independent of services is linked to finance and employment. Remaining in employment for some

HPs is an attempt to 'continue as normal'. For others it is an economic necessity. Only two HPs were in paid employment at the time of the interview. These HPs highlighted the inflexibility of services for employed, asymptomatic HPs. One had been forced to take holiday time off work in order to attend the clinic for a regular check up as he did not want to inform his employers of his status. Eventually he tackled the clinic about their inaccessible opening times and they agreed to see him by special arrangement.

Another HP who was obliged to visit the hospital every fortnight for medication found that his appointments frequently coincided with work times. He was unable to afford the equipment to administer his medication at home. But, when he applied for a grant, he was told that he was not (in his words) 'suitably ill' because he was working.

Claiming benefits

Five of the six HPs, and one informal carer, said that their financial situation had been very much affected by the HP's health status. The other informal carers described their financial situation as largely unaffected, but this was perhaps because they were receiving benefits or sick pay due to their own ill health.

There was general agreement amongst HPs and informal carers that information about availability and entitlement to benefits was sparse, and that making a claim was exhausting and demoralizing. One informal carer said of her son's claim for invalidity benefit:

It was made so awkward we nearly didn't bother. (IC3)

She then described the assessment procedure which was designed to 'prove' his disability.

He was told to walk unaided. I was so afraid that he would fall and hurt himself, and lose his dignity. It really should have been sufficient to have the doctor's signature. (IC3)

Ironically, it took so long for the benefit application to be processed that he only received one payment before he died.

One relatively asymptomatic HP felt justified in lying to get benefits, as necessary preparation for his future ill health.

I try to work in advance to set up help because it's too stressful to fight when you are ill. (HP2)

Financial independence was not just viewed in practical terms but was equated with psychological independence and a desire for 'normality'. For example, one HP was worried that he might lose his house and have to go into care for financial reasons, losing associations with memories of his partner as well as personal independence.

Self-help and control

All respondents noted the importance of self-help and stress reduction strategies. It is commonly believed that stress plays an important part in the conversion from being asymptomatic to ill health, and must therefore be minimized. One preventative strategy identified by HPs and informal carers was affordable and accessible complementary therapies.

> There is a definite need for the use of alternative therapy. If you can't cure us, the least you can do is to make us feel comfortable. (HP1)

Perceived benefits included stress reduction, physical comfort, 'time out' and 'recharging the batteries'. But, perhaps most importantly:

> They make you feel that you are doing something for yourself. (HP3)

The feeling of being in control of the illness, and of care, seems to become more important, but less attainable, the longer a person has HIV. 'Healthy' choices may become more and more restricted by financial circumstances as the disease progresses. One HP explained that, since becoming ill, he found it necessary to spend an increasing amount of his meagre income on heating his house. There is little hope of controlling the progression of HIV if, for example, choices have to be made between keeping warm and eating. Such dilemmas themselves are a major source of worry, further restricting control over ill health.

HIV as a chronic illness

The chronic nature of HIV takes its toll on HPs, informal carers and service providers, financially, mentally, physically and emotionally.

The financial drain associated with HIV is exacerbated by the inability of many HPs and informal carers to continue to work, difficulty in obtaining benefits and increased expenditure required to travel out of the local area to obtain services. For example, one HP, who felt it necessary to use services in a neighbouring city because of the perceived inadequacy of local services, reported that his visits were restricted by lack of money.

> I like going there. It's really helpful, but some weeks I have to cancel my appointments because I can't afford to get there. (HP6)

Ironically, when he arrived at the clinic, his travel expenses were refunded.

One consultant, who was aware of the detrimental effect of long term poverty on patients' health, felt justified in admitting a patient to hospital for a few days respite. This is an example of an acute sector provider 'filling the gap' in community service provision, and was only possible because of the low prevalence of HIV in the area. It is also an example of a cost-ineffective and reactive measure.

Call for specific HIV services

HPs and service providers complained about their lack of knowledge of HIV and of local HIV service provision. Respondents criticized testing and follow-up treatment in genito-urinary clinics. Several HPs were concerned about confidentiality amongst GPs. One HP was disconcerted by the possibility of being treated at the local hospital, as the ward most commonly used by HIV patients comes under the chest physician.

> The first thing I noticed about Ward X was that it was full of geri-atrics. I might catch something there. AIDS wards are less conta-gious. (HP3)

HPs and service providers alike called for the development of HIV-specific services as a way of improving service standards. HPs indicated that they would welcome the convenience and greater expertise that this would encourage. Service providers wanted specialist colleagues with sufficient time and interest to provide a quality service, but felt that this would only happen when they were unable to provide even an adequate service.

> We need a specialist-led service.... It may be that, in 10 years time, we will have so many people that we will need an HIV consultant. We'll only get one when we can't cope with the demand by filling the gaps. (Consultant 4)

The limitations of HIV services in North Yorkshire place increasing pressures on key HIV service providers. Their expertise and personal commitment are maintaining the existing system and obscuring the need to develop services. At the same time, HPs are placing more demands on certain service providers and forcing them into a 'key worker' role. The stress that this places on the service provider, coupled with inadequate support from the system, increases the likelihood of service provider burnout and further weakens the system.

HPs appreciated the commitment of particular service providers.

> If it wasn't for [community HIV worker] I would be very isolated. She always makes time, and makes us feel very comfortable. (HP1)

The same HP expressed anxiety about being let down if he became too reliant on services.

> I would like reassurance of continuity of services. One of my fears is that, when I'm very ill, I'm not sure the services will be there for me.

It's very difficult for us to trust and build relationships, and this is not helped if they're not going to be there six months later. (HP1)

Deciding whether to accept help was a 'wicked problem' (see Introduction) for him because, by accepting help, he became dependent and so vulnerable to being let down.

DISCUSSION

The research findings, admittedly from a small sample of HPs and informal carers, suggest that HIV services in North Yorkshire are generally uncoordinated, reactive and uninformed by experience. They are held together through the commitment of a few key individuals. Many providers are aware of the inadequacies of their services and attribute them to the lack of support by purchasers and the low local prevalence of HIV. HPs, angered by these inadequacies, are either voting with their feet or increasing their demands on the few people who can provide the service they require.

Purchasers should note that, unlike many service users, people with HIV are motivated and have the opportunity to seek out excellence. Service users want improvements in the standards of local services and see the development of specific HIV services as the way forward. It is to be hoped that research recommendations will inform purchasing decisions. But there can be no guarantees, even when, as with the present study, it was commissioned by purchasers.

CHAPTER 13

The rise and fall of a self-help support project

Susan J. Milner and Don Watson

INTRODUCTION

In 1987 an innovative project, designed to promote health through the provision of support for self-help activities, was opened in a large town which is one of the most deprived in the North of England. The project was initiated by the Health Promotion Department of the local District Health Authority.

This chapter describes the establishment, operation and demise of the project. The main focus of the chapter is work undertaken with local self-help groups to establish user perspectives on the development of the project. Two studies are described. One used questionnaires, and the other focused discussions, to explore with self-help group members the value to them personally of group membership, and of the project, in supporting local self-help activity. The chapter concludes with a discussion of the changing organizational backdrop to the project which ultimately contributed to its closure.

Self-help and community development

The greater prevalence of ill health and so called 'at risk' behaviours in social classes IV and V have long been a challenge to health promoters. Those most in need of health promotion seem to benefit least from what has traditionally been offered, e.g. advice from health professionals, mass media campaigns. Such efforts threaten to widen the health gap between social groups and alternative approaches have been sought (Gatherer *et al.*, 1980). Members of social classes IV and V have been found to be more likely to respond positively to interpersonal forms of communication, especially from credible people within their own community (Friedson, 1961; Rodgers and Shoemaker, 1971).

In response, health promoters became interested in community based initiatives characterized by informality, lay participation, an emphasis on reducing social disadvantage in health and an overall aim of 'empowering' individuals to make 'informed choices' about their health (Tones, Tilford and Robinson, 1990).

Such initiatives are associated with the philosophy of community development, an approach which claims to recognize and challenge social and political barriers to good health (Gulbenkian Foundation, 1968; Hubley, 1980). Community development is about working in and with communities to stimulate them to identify and articulate their own needs, and to support them in collective action to meet those needs

This approach de-emphasizes lifestyle as the focal point for health promotion, claiming that it leads to 'victim-blaming' and that it ignores more powerful determinants of health, such as sociopolitical factors that lead to multiple disadvantage and poverty (Townsend and Davidson, 1982; Tudor Hart, 1971; Whitehead, 1987; Townsend, Phillimore and Beattie, 1988).

'Self-help' is an important element in the community development approach, as it provides one way in which individuals can take more control over their own health experience and redefine the issues for themselves. Tension between self-help groups and health care professionals can result from the required shift in the balance of power between these two parties (Hatch and Kickbusch, 1983).

The nature of self-help

Self-help groups vary enormously in composition and focus. Katz and Bender (1976) have described self-help groups as coming together voluntarily for mutual aid and the accomplishment of a special purpose. They are often set up by individuals who feel that their needs are not, or cannot be, met by existing social institutions. Groups may provide material assistance as well as emotional support, and their activities may centre on a specific 'problem'. They usually foster an ideology or set of values through which members may obtain an enhanced sense of personal identity.

In order to see how self-help might contribute to the promotion of health it is useful to distinguish three levels of health promotion.

- Primary health promotion aims to prevent well people from becoming ill.
- Secondary health promotion is targeted at those who may be displaying early symptoms or have a reversible problem. The aim here is to restore health and prevent recurrence.
- Tertiary health promotion aims to maximize the quantity and quality of life of people who have a permanent health problem or terminal illness.

Self-help groups can contribute at all three levels. Some groups have primary health promotion as their main purpose, e.g. women's health groups. Others may meet because they are trying to deal with a common health problem, e.g. diabetes or asthma, and so are mainly involved in secondary or tertiary health promotion.

The potential benefits of self-help group membership are not confined to participants. The groups can stimulate changes in statutory service provision and educational activities for professionals. Informal carers of people who participate because they have a health problem may also benefit directly or indirectly from such activity, often at a very practical level, for example, obtaining advice on welfare benefits or respite care.

Supporting self-help

By definition, self-help is something people do for themselves, rather than something they have done to them by paid workers. However, self-help group participation can be very demanding, especially for group leaders, where they exist. Setting up a new group or running/joining an established one requires confidence and social and organizational skill. Meeting rooms, refreshments, administrative support and other practical necessities are not automatically available within the group. There is a strong case for making it easier to initiate and develop self-help groups by providing a degree of practical support.

Delbecq and Van der Ven (1971) have argued that self-help groups can encourage cathartic exchanges and discourage people from challenging the root cause of the problem. As such, they could be used by professionals to control and manipulate clients. The independent status of some self-help groups can be compromised by contact with outside 'support' agencies. Even peripheral or sensitively handled contact can, potentially, lead to outside 'interference', as can attempts to investigate user perspectives. Researchers need to be aware of this dilemma and to be able to justify their activities in terms of overall gain for the groups concerned.

The project

The project was located in a town centre, shop front, 'drop in' health information centre. It was open during extended office hours, four days per week, and was available to clients outside these hours for a range of health promotion activities.

The project catered to a wide range of clients, and had two main functions:

- to provide free, confidential, accurate information and advice to members of the public on a wide range of health-related topics and

services; this information was offered on a 'drop in' or telephone enquiry basis by a trained health promotion specialist;
- to support local self-help activity by working to meet the needs of existing groups or individuals wanting to set up a new group, with support tailored to meet the needs of each group.

The focus of this chapter is on the second of these functions, self-help support. The next section describes two pieces of empirical work, using questionnaires and focus groups, which were undertaken with self-help clients in order to determine their expressed needs and guide service provision.

THE SELF-HELP GROUP SURVEY

Methods

In 1991, a survey of local self-help groups was carried out. The survey aimed to investigate the benefits which members saw in participation, and the support which they felt that their group needed.

The survey consisted of a self-completed postal questionnaire. Only part of the first section, covering the benefits of membership of the self-help group and the need for support, will be discussed in this chapter. The questions, which are outlined in the Results section, provided a list of likely answers, established in exploratory work, which respondents were invited to agree or disagree with, and an open section for 'other' replies.

The questionnaire was piloted twice before final administration (each pilot sample $n = 10$).

The sample

Sampling self-help groups

It was not possible to obtain a truly representative random sample of self-help group members or groups. In general, such groups are not highly visible or accessible organizations. Many are not listed anywhere, and contact can only be made through community networks.

The sample obtained for this research could be described as an 'incomplete population sample'. There was no way of knowing the exact number of self-help groups functioning within the boundaries of the area covered by the health authority as many were small and very locally based. Groups emerge and disappear quickly. However, the project built up an up-to-date and comprehensive catalogue of local self-help groups and other organizations offering health-related services to the community. From that catalogue, approximately 150 local self-help groups could be identified. They covered a wide variety of topic areas and varied a great deal in structure and function. About 50 of the groups were already in contact with the project.

The 150 groups were listed alphabetically and every alternate group was selected for inclusion in the sample. Of the 75 groups approached, 49 (65%) agreed to take part. In some cases, the initial point of contact led to more than one self-help group. Eventually, 56 groups, with a total membership of 876 individuals, were included in the sample. A further seven groups decided to withdraw, mainly because of anticipated difficulties in questionnaire distribution by the group contact. This reduced the number of groups to 49 with a total membership of 623.

There were no obvious differences in the aims of the 49 groups who eventually participated and the 26 who did not. However, non-participant groups may have differed in other ways, e.g. cohesiveness, quality of organization.

Method of administration

The researcher negotiated with the contact person for each of the groups included in the sample either to deliver the required number of questionnaires to them for distribution (the majority of cases), or to post the questionnaires out to group members from address lists supplied by the contact person. Stamped addressed envelopes were supplied with the questionnaire for return. Follow up reminder letters were sent to each contact person four and eight weeks after the initial distribution date of the questionnaire.

Response rates

Of the 623 questionnaires sent out, 318 (51%) were completed and returned by self-help group members from 42 groups. No questionnaires were returned from seven groups and it seems likely that they were not distributed by the contact person. No obvious common theme linked these groups.

Results

The perceived benefits of being in a self-help group

Respondents were asked about the benefits they saw in membership of a self-help group. A total of 12 benefits previously highlighted by group members during the development of the questionnaire were listed, and respondents were asked to state whether or not they felt that these applied to themselves. In addition, there was an open section, allowing respondents to add any further benefits or comments if they wished. Responses are summarized in Table 13.1.

Table 13.1 The benefits of being in a self-help group as perceived by group members ($n = 318$)

Benefit	%	n
Speaking to others in the same boat	83.0	264
Don't feel so alone with my problem	80.2	255
Friendship/companionship	73.6	234
Able to share my problems	73.0	232
More access to information	68.2	217
Practical advice	64.8	206
Social outlet	56.9	181
Access to practical help or extra services	46.5	148
Feel more in control	38.7	123
More self-confident	37.7	120
Better able to make decision	30.8	98
More able to deal with professionals	27.0	86
Other stated benefits (open section)	9.7	31

The main perceived benefits of belonging to a self-help group involved sharing the 'problem', information and advice and being with others in a similar situation. Friendship/companionship and providing a social outlet were each mentioned by more than half the sample. Benefits relating to feeling more confident, in control or able to make decisions were also highlighted by respondents, but not to the same extent.

Support required by self-help groups

Self-help groups are generally run by members for the benefit of members, but they do sometimes receive help from others, e.g. health or social care professionals, national headquarters or other voluntary groups. When asked if their group had ever needed outside help, but did not receive it, 28.6% (91) answered 'yes'. Of these individuals, 42% (38) belonged to groups which had asked for and been refused help, 31% (28) had not known whom to ask and 16% (15) decided not to ask.

Respondents were asked to state when, if at all, their group had been helped by an outside agent, and the nature of that help. The results are summarized in Table 13.2.

Respondents were asked to remember past events concerning support for the group. It is possible, therefore, that the figures in Table 13.2 under-estimate the extent to which groups had requested support. A substantial minority did not know whether their group had sought help. However, about half the sample indicated that their group had requested outside help when setting up, and a similar proportion stated that their group had done so since it had become established. This result suggests that groups need ongoing support that extends beyond the difficult period of getting a new group off the ground.

Table 13.2   Nature of outside support for self-help groups (n = 318)

Outside help used	% yes (n)	% no (n)	% DK (n)
When group was setting up	44.6 (142)	19.5 (62)	35.9 (114)
After group established	55.3 (176)	23.3 (74)	21.4 (68)

Source of help	%	n
Health worker (e.g. doctor, nurse)	46.8	117
National HQ (if any)	25.2	80
Voluntary agencies	15.4	49
Community worker	14.8	47
Social worker	12.6	40
Community Health Council	9.4	30
Other source (open section)	5.0	16

Type of help	%	n
Attracting new members	34.0	109
Advice on publicity	32.7	104
Typing/photocopying	30.5	97
Leaflet and poster production	27.7	88
Advice on funds	27.4	87
Advice on accommodation	26.7	85
Advice on getting speakers	26.7	85
Discussing ideas or problems about group	24.8	79
Facilitating contact with professionals	24.2	77
Facilitating contact with other groups	21.1	67
A contact point for mail/phone calls	20.4	65
Help with transport	18.2	58
Help with training (e.g. health-related)	13.9	44
Advice on how to run meetings	12.6	40
Sorting out disagreements or group dynamics	9.5	30
Other (open section)	2.1	7

Sources of support for self-help groups

Table 13.2 shows that the most common sources of support were health workers (e.g. doctors, nurses, health visitors) and national headquarters. Only 64.5% (205) of respondents belonged to groups which were affiliated to national headquarters, and 39% (80) of members of these groups stated that they had received help from HQ. National headquarters were thus mentioned most frequently as a source of support by members of affiliated groups.

Other sources of help which, by the nature of their roles, might have been expected to be prominent sources of support, were mentioned by 15% of the sample or less. These included community and social workers, Community Health Councils and voluntary agencies such as Councils for Voluntary Service.

These results may reflect no more than the relative numbers of individuals employed in these different roles. Because health care workers are so numerous, in comparison with the other groups, it is not surprising that they emerged as the most important source of support. However, their training and orientation would not necessarily make them the most appropriate people to meet the expressed needs of members of self-help groups, e.g. for organizational assistance.

Types of support

Table 13.2 shows that self-help groups received a wide range of types of support, mostly involving assistance with administration and recruitment of new members.

The Self-Help Support Project provided assistance in all the categories highlighted in the survey as being important to groups apart from help with transport. A similar range of needs was identified in the second, focus group, study discussed in the next section.

THE SELF-HELP FOCUS GROUPS STUDY

Introduction

As part of the research into the needs of self-help groups, a qualitative, exploratory study was undertaken in 1992 with members of seven selected self-help groups. The research explored a number of questions.

- Had being in the group affected their self-confidence?
- Did they value themselves more?
- Did they feel more able to make decisions?
- Did they feel more in control or did they feel dependent on the group?
- What forms of external support did the groups feel they needed?

Methods

To explore these issues, in-depth focus group discussions were used. Focus group discussions bring together six to eight respondents with particular knowledge of the research topic under the guidance of a group moderator. This is a small enough number for everyone to share insights, and large enough for a diverse range of perceptions. Respondents typically do not know each other (Mendes de Almeida, 1980; Tynan and Drayton, 1988) but have homogeneous characteristics that encourage them to feel more at ease with each other. They might, for example, be of a similar age, socioeconomic group, sex, or of similar marital status.

Group moderation is based on the principle that each participant is encouraged to express his/her views and is exposed to the views of fellow group members.

After introducing herself, the moderator (SM) explained that the discussion was to be about the group they belonged to, that she was interested in **their** experiences and thoughts and that there were no right or wrong answers. The tape recorder was introduced at this point.

The 'funnel technique' was used (Krueger, 1988). Respondents were asked general questions while rapport was being established during the first 10–15 minutes, followed by more specific questions when the atmosphere was relaxed. A discussion guide, memorized prior to moderation, was used. The discussions lasted 60–90 minutes and were taped with respondents' permission. The tape recorder was placed out of sight to make it less inhibiting. Respondents were assured of confidentiality and that the recorder was being used as a memory aid. The atmosphere in the focus groups was mostly relaxed, friendly and personal although there was more participant involvement in some sessions than in others.

There is no right or wrong way to analyse and interpret qualitative data (Market Research Society, 1979; Basch, 1987; Tynan and Drayton, 1988; Robson and Foster, 1989). In this case, the moderator transcribed the tapes and collated the relevant information under headings describing the issues which emerged. Quotations have been used to illustrate the findings.

The sample

Because of the nature of the research topic, respondents were recruited as a preformed group. Normally, in focus group discussions, members should not know each other, for two reasons. Firstly, acquaintances are more likely to begin talking in a 'split off' subgroup. Secondly, inhibitions can be heightened if members feel that they are being judged by people whom they know outside the group. It can also be useful to observe how groups 'bond' during the discussion.

In the present research, members of the groups knew each other and some 'bonding' had already taken place. This did enable the dynamics of each self-help group to be observed. However, because the majority of the respondents were regular attenders, they were less likely to have negative attitudes and opinions about the self-help group to which they belonged, potentially biasing the results.

The following groups were recruited:

- Women's Health Group;
- Anxiety and Depression Group;
- Over 50s Friendship Group;
- Carers of Alzheimer Sufferers Luncheon Club;

- Loss Support Group;
- Epileptics Support Group;
- Young Mothers and Toddlers Group.

These groups were selected on the basis of ease of access, variety of group type and relationship with the project. Usually, about 50–70% of the members of selected groups chose to attend the focus groups.

Results

The benefits of being in a self-help group

The perceived benefits of being in a self-help group can be summarized under a number of headings.

Self-confidence
Many participants had experienced a change in their personal circumstances, e.g. bereavement or divorce, and felt trapped in a cycle in which loss of self-confidence made it hard for them to go out and not going out reduced their self-confidence.

> I think when you're bereaved you lose all your confidence, for a time anyway. (Over 50s Friendship Group)

The support and encouragement they gained from other group members helped them to build up self-confidence.

> I'm more confident now when I go out. I can speak out now. I couldn't before I lost my husband, because he took all the reins off me. (Over 50s Friendship Group)

The problem identified by the above person was not the bereavement as such but the change which it caused in her wider relationships with the community, previously managed by her husband.

Self-esteem
People who had been isolated because of an illness sometimes experienced feelings of low self-esteem and worthlessness.

> The tension and anxiety and depression, agoraphobia, whatever, can get that bad that you don't want to go on. (Anxiety Group)

> Death's got to be better. (Anxiety Group)

Participating in a group could help, because people learnt that their problems were not unique.

> I really did think, like all of us thought, I was the only one that could possibly be suffering. (Epilepsy Group)

Ability to cope
Belonging to a group helped members to feel that they could cope with the symptoms of their illness, their situation and other people.

> [Being in the group means] ... they won't feel guilty being ill. (Epilepsy Group)

Practical advice was also needed.

> After this thing is diagnosed ... no-one can tell you what to apply for, and what you can get. No-one gives you any information. You have to find out for yourself. (Carers of Alzheimer Sufferers)

By sharing their experiences, group members could give and receive such advice.

> One chap says to me, 'How do you get your wife's tights on?'... Or X will say, 'You want to get a seat for the bath.' (Carers of Alzheimer Sufferers)

Respite from stress was an important benefit for some.

> I can come here on me own, and it's absolutely fantastic. Whether it sounds harsh to you or not, I don't know, but to me it's fantastic to get away for a few hours. (Carers of Alzheimer Sufferers)

> [It's like] time out. (Women's Health Group)

> Sometimes you need something for yourself. (Women's Health Group)

Participating in a group helped informal carers to cope with their roles.

> And when you get back [to caree] you're a better person because you've had your batteries recharged. (Carers of Alzheimer Sufferers)

Control
Improved self-confidence had led many to feel more positive about themselves, and, as a result, to feel more in control of their lives.

> I was stuck in the house every day. Then I came here [anxiety group] one night. Then, gradually, from then on, I started to go out. (Anxiety Group)

Relationships and social lives
Some felt that they had become more aware of other people, and were less bound up in themselves. Talking with other group members and asking questions of others had helped to shift the focus from themselves.

Now I've become more loving, you know, and touchy [willing to touch] which I was never before, and I think that's just associated with coming here. (Anxiety Group)

Some participants established relationships with other members outside the group, or were able to develop social activities independently, because they felt they had become more cheerful, motivated, enthusiastic and positive.

From meeting here we've formed friendships that carry on outside the club. (Over 50s Friendship Group)

Interactions with health and social services

Those in the disease related groups had sometimes had difficult experiences with health professionals and the social services.

There's no information in the form of a leaflet or even one person who has all the information so the carer can ring up and ask. (Carers of Alzheimer Sufferers)

Many expressed anger at the unsatisfactory way they had been treated.

Somebody should come to you, not you to them. (Epilepsy Group)

Health professionals were seen as often lacking in knowledge and experience of the specific problem which the group was concerned with.

I think that general practitioners and quite a number of consultants are not far enough up with dementia. (Carers of Alzheimer Sufferers)

Those who had had good experiences mostly felt that they had been lucky. A minority had been willing to battle to get the care that they wanted.

I felt as if all the way along the line I've had to fight the medical profession. (Anxiety Group)

Some talked about feeling belittled or disempowered in dealing, for example, with social services, partly because they did not know how the system worked, but also because they detected a 'them and us' attitude. Some had been put off using services, and only did so with the encouragement of group members.

The self-help group as a community

Belonging to a self-help group enabled members to be part of a community, as defined in Chapter 1. They could identify with a group which had similarities of experience and outlook *vis à vis* the outside world, and attempt to sustain collective but personal autonomy of action. The support provided by self-help groups therefore has inherent advantages over that given by formal carers or volunteer 'friends' (Chapter 11).

Group support needs

Although the support needs for each of the groups differed, there were some common themes.

Finance

The need for financial support, large or small, was mentioned by five of the seven groups. Substantial financial support was required by one group because it was part of a community house under threat of closure (later in 1992) due to insufficient funds.

> Without the house all the groups are going to go anyway. So we've all got to raise money for the house. (Women's Health Group)

The Anxiety Group needed a small sum to improve conditions at their weekly meetings.

> We find that if we do our relaxation in these chairs, that are so hard, they can't relax their bodies. (Anxiety Group)

The Self-Help Support Project was able to offer small amounts of money to groups, usually in the form of start-up grants, and to provide a range of direct support services, e.g. postage, telephone, duplicating, typing and accommodation, reducing the need for some groups to raise funds. For those groups who did seek to raise funds, the project offered support in preparing applications.

Transport

Lack of transport prevented some potential members of the groups from being able to participate.

> If I had transport I could have sent for him, brought him here, and could have him in the group. (Anxiety Group)

The project was not able to offer a transport service, but it did access a local free community transport service whenever possible. This arrangement was less than satisfactory for groups meeting out of office hours.

Accommodation

Three of the seven groups used the accommodation provided by the project. The Over 50s Friendship Group was very settled and secure in its running. None of the participants raised the issue of support. However, they were grateful for the use of the room in the Health Information Centre, and, before the sudden closure of the project, could not see anything that might jeopardize their position!

In addition to the rooms at the centre the project had free access to other accommodation in the town centre. It was also possible to obtain access to health authority premises or to pay for accommodation on behalf of a group on a time-limited basis.

New recruits
Participants sought help in encouraging new members to attend. One of the main roles of the self-help support project was to assist with recruitment, not just in the initial phase of a group's life, but whenever needed.

Leadership backup
In one group, participants felt strongly that the leader needed support in the form of a stand-in who could run the group if she was unable to.

> I think too much is left on [leader]. There's not enough help....
> [Leader] is a sufferer ... and, therefore, there may be a time when
> she might feel that it's too much to come to the group. (Anxiety
> Group)

Speakers
Speakers were seen to play a useful role in stimulating the group, giving them things to talk about, helping them to bond in the early stages, and providing new insights and experiences. Participants in one group felt they were running out of ideas for outside speakers.

The project was able to assist, using the wide network of local and national contacts it had established, both within and outside the NHS, and was able to pay for some speakers.

Members of the Alzheimer's Disease Carers Luncheon Club were angry that they had had little advice, in written form or from health professionals and the social services, about the symptoms of the disease, what to expect and the benefits they were entitled to. Help was suggested here in the form of outside speakers who were empathetic, knew what they were talking about and were experienced in caring.

Improved relationship with professionals
Being part of the NHS enabled project workers frequently to act as go-betweens or advocates for groups, not just with health professionals but with other statutory and non-statutory organizations. For example, they arranged appointments with managers and clinicians and acted as advocates for the groups at planning meetings.

Conversely, there were occasions when it was not possible for the project to become overtly involved in some of the groups' activities, e.g. complaints about service reductions or lack of services, because of the real or potential disapproval of the health authority.

DISCUSSION

Research implications

The results of the focus group discussions confirmed the conclusion of the questionnaire survey, that the groups found the services offered by the Self-Help Support Project both useful and necessary in varying degrees.

Taken together, the results would suggest that the project had been successful in identifying the needs of its client group, and in directing service provision towards meeting those needs, within resource and organizational limits. The research also showed that the needs of individual groups changed over time, and that the project, therefore, needed to remain flexible in its approach to self-help support. Initially, groups frequently wanted help with setting up and recruitment. As they became established, groups often needed assistance in developing their activities, e.g. getting speakers, going on training courses. Established groups sometimes needed help with group dynamic problems.

Organizational background to the project

This project was an attempt by the Health Promotion Department of the District Health Authority to make health promotion services more accessible and acceptable to residents of the town. It was funded for an initial period of three years by the Government's Urban Programme. It was managed on a day-to-day basis by a project manager, but was an integral part of the Health Promotion Department. The work of the project formed part of this department's operational plan, agreed with the General Manager of the Community Unit to which the department belonged.

These managerial arrangements continued until the introduction of the NHS and Community Care Act 1990. This legislation fundamentally altered the structure of the NHS by transforming the role of the District Health Authority (DHA). The DHA had previously owned and managed all NHS facilities and services within its geographical boundary. The new legislation introduced the concept of the purchaser/provider split. The DHA became responsible for assessing the health needs of their resident population, and for purchasing services to meet those needs from appropriate providers. The DHA lost management responsibility for hospitals and community services units, which became independent providers of services under contract to a possible range of purchasers.

Because the Self-Help Support Project was part of the Health Promotion Department, which was itself part of the Community Services Unit, it became a provider of services under the new arrangements. The funding of the project didn't change, as the Government's Urban Programme renewed financial support on two occasions (an unusual occurrence within this local authority). However, the money was awarded to the Health Authority, not the Community Services Unit to which the project belonged.

The 1991/2 contract between the DHA and the Community Services Unit included 'self-help support', but it was not considered a priority by the purchaser, who thought that it was a job for the Social Services Department. The 1992/3 contract did not include 'self-help support'. Purchaser commitment to public health information continued, but was tied in with the condition that there would be a collaborative health information project with the Family Health Services Authority (FHSA). A new joint information centre was to be commissioned by 1994, and the existing project closed.

In August 1992 the project was closed. Users were given up to a month's notice of withdrawal of services. The Community Health Council, which has a statutory right to be consulted over proposed reductions in services, was not consulted, only given two weeks notice of the closure. Those groups in regular contact with the project were told one month in advance. At the time of closure, 15 groups were using the project as their only meeting place. Six were found alternative accommodation.

The Self-Help Support Project successfully employed user perspectives research to demonstrate that it was meeting their needs and as a guide to service development. However, in the new NHS world of the purchaser/provider split, this research did not influence purchasing decisions. The contracts managers of the Community Services Unit were either unable or unwilling to press for this service to be included in the contract.

This example should illustrate to all those involved in project management, research and evaluation the need for timely and 'manager-friendly' presentation of results. Projects which meet user needs, particularly community development initiatives which take a long time to root and show obvious results, will be lost unless purchasers are able to see how they will contribute to the achievement of their strategic aims.

CHAPTER 14

From the hospital to community health care: Foucauldian analyses

Sarah Nettleton

INTRODUCTION

In the early 19th century, formal medical care was primarily concerned with diseased bodies, which were most suitably treated within the domain of the hospital. By contrast, contemporary health and medical care is dispersed throughout multiple locations and involves the maintenance and the promotion of health throughout the community.

This chapter aims to examine the shift from hospital to community. It does this by drawing upon and reviewing a body of literature that is explicitly Foucauldian (Nettleton and Burrows, 1994). Over the last decade a growing number of researchers have drawn upon the work of Foucault and in so doing have provided alternative ways of understanding and accounting for social and organizational puzzles. One such puzzle is: why in western liberal democracies has the provision of health care for a range of patient groups such as the mentally ill, people with learning difficulties, the elderly and the chronically ill been found to be more appropriate in the community than in relatively isolated institutions? A second but not unrelated question is: what are the conditions that have permitted the analysis of the views of users of community health services and interpretations of their experience of health and health care?

Thus the aims of this chapter are, boldly stated, the complexities and discussions concerning boundaries, meanings and definitions that are to some extent submerged by the polarity of hospital versus community. However, these debates are rehearsed in Chapter 1. This chapter aims to offer a more 'removed' analysis of general trends in health care, rather than becoming immersed in contemporary political and theoretical battles about the merits or appropriateness of various forms of health care. While those studies that have adopted Foucault's genealogical methodology (Armstrong, 1990; Nettleton, 1992) examine in detail the mundane routines of everyday life, their intentions are to illuminate more fundamental discursive transformations. More specifically, they aim to explore the differential ways in which bodies are regulated, understood and constructed by researchers and practitioners. In practice, this involves listening to professionals, reading through journals and observing the activities of practitioners.

What unifies the studies reviewed in this chapter is the idea that the objects of the medical or social sciences are an effect of the practices that surround them. Thus, the chapters in this volume that describe or evaluate the consumer's perspective have contributed to the fabrication of an active and vocal patient, user or client. If we are to understand changes in the organization of health and medical care we must begin by exploring how the objects of its focus are constructed.

The prime object of medical care located within the hospital was a diseased anatomy. The central object of health care located in the community is a 'whole person' who simultaneously manifests a potential to be ill and a potential to be increasingly healthy. Moreover the whole person has a voice, a view and a valid perspective, which is now regarded as a crucial dimension of effective health care. The need to listen to patients is central to the reformed National Health Service (NHS), as the NHS Management Executive (NHSME, 1993b) are keen to point out: 'Consumer satisfaction in the health service means much more than the occasional patient satisfaction survey, although these have their place. It means replacing "we know best" by "you know best". It means systematically involving patients in planning services, reviewing their effectiveness and even, where possible, in the actual process of care' (p. 6).

Thus the consumer's perspective has become established in the rhetoric, at least, of contemporary health care.

In order to realize the aim of this chapter, I will attempt to achieve four objectives. Firstly, I will introduce those aspects of Foucault's work that have influenced studies of health care. In particular, I will draw attention to the fact that the rise of pathological medicine was instrumental for the foundation of other related human sciences. Secondly, I will discuss Armstrong's work on the reconfiguration of medical knowledge in Britain in the 20th century and how this contributed to the construction of the patient as a whole person within the context of the community. Thirdly, I will take one example of an area of health care, namely psychiatric care, to illustrate in more detail the social processes involved in the transition from hospital to community care. Finally I will briefly allude to a transformation that western health care systems are currently experiencing.

THE WORK OF FOUCAULT: BODIES AND DISCIPLINES

Two aspects of Foucault's work have particularly influenced analyses of health care and are of significance to the present discussion. The first is the notion that ways of looking at and examining the body construct its reality. The second is that power within modern societies has become more diffuse and has moved from the central location of the state or sovereign to a multiplicity of sites throughout the society.

In *The Birth of the Clinic*, Foucault (1976), like many other historians (e.g. Ackerknecht, 1967), describes how, at the turn of the 18th century, a specific notion of disease emerged along with the development of the pathological anatomy. The classificatory medicine (i.e. the classification of diseases into types) that had existed for centuries before gave way to the anatomo-clinical method, the 'scientific' biomedicine that we know today. Disease came to be formulated as a discrete phenomenon which was located within the workings of the bodily structures.

What distinguishes Foucault's account is that he sees this conceptualization of disease as an effect of what he calls '*le regard*', which has been translated as 'the gaze'. The gaze is a 'way of seeing' (or indeed, smelling or touching). It was through the medical gaze that things became visible to the physician and, once formulated as discrete entities, could be observed and analysed. Thus, at the end of the 18th century, there was a change in the relationship between what could be seen and what could be said. Truth came to reside in the empirical look. The medical gaze was not a static way of looking. On the contrary, its flexibility, as we shall see, constantly permitted new objects to come in to view.

Foucault locates this change in the context of teaching hospitals which were established in Paris after the French Revolution. The new medicine came about because it was taught in the hospital ward rather than the lecture theatre. It was in the former that the origin of truth lay. Patients, or bodies, became the object of scientific knowledge and practice. The truth about illness and disease lay in the interior of the body. Indeed medicine could only ever be absolutely certain about disease once the patient had died and the body could be dissected. This explains the prime importance that is given to the dissection of a body when medical students embark on their careers. 'Nineteenth century medicine was haunted by that absolute eye that cadaverizes life and rediscovers in the corpse the frail, broken nervure of life' (Foucault, 1976, p. 166).

Thus the teaching hospital formed the prerequisite to 'the birth of the clinic', as here doctors derived their knowledge from what they could see rather than what they read in books. The gaze formed a kind of 'language without words ... a language that did not owe its truth to speech but to the gaze alone' (Foucault, 1976, p. 68–9).

What is significant for our argument here is that the body is a product of the discourse in which it is located. It is an effect of the techniques of analysis that surround and pervade it. As Prior (1989) succinctly explains: 'A discourse, moreover, is not merely a narrow set of linguistic practices which reports on the world, but is composed of a whole assemblage of activities, events, objects, settings and epistemological percepts' (p. 3). It was within the discursive context of modern institutions such as the teaching hospital and the prison that the individual came to be an object of scientific knowledge, giving rise to what we now know as the human sciences. Likewise, and more recently, it is within the discursive context of the community that the active and participating patient was found.

The centrality of the body to all the human sciences is a theme that was further perused by Foucault (1979) in *Discipline and Punish: The Birth of the Prison*. This book is not simply a history of the penal system. It is 'a genealogy of the present scientifico-legal complex from which the power to punish deserves its bases,... a specific mode of subjection was able to give birth to man [sic] as an object of knowledge for a discourse with a scientific status' (pp. 23-4). At the same time that the body was discovered in the hospital, it was imprisoned in the penitentiary. In both cases, bodies were located into institutional sites where they could be observed, analysed, understood and assessed. They were subjected to surveillance. It was these techniques of surveillance that engendered our scientific knowledge of them. This is what is meant by the concept **power/knowledge**.

Power, in the sense of disciplinary power, refers to those techniques and activities that work upon the body which in turn yield knowledge of it. Our knowledge of the body is always circumscribed. It is an effect of the means that are employed to analyse it. In the 19th century, the main sites of surveillance, or disciplinary power, were institutions such as the hospital, the prison, the school and the military camp.

Foucault found the ideal representation of power in the design of Bentham's Panopticon. The Panopticon was a peripheral design in which cells surrounded a central tower. This facilitated the perpetual observation of the inmates, and, more importantly, induced the inmates to watch over and monitor their own behaviour. That people monitor their own behaviour is regarded by Foucault as one of the central elements of modern society. The inducement to be aware of our actions began within institutions, and has now become more diffused throughout society.

PANOPTIC TO DISPENSARY POWER

The advent of the 20th century witnessed a shift in the diagram of power. The exterior walls of the Panopticon began to crumble. Disciplinary power has increasingly infiltrated the community. This is explored within the context of medicine by Armstrong (1983) in his seminal book *The Political Anatomy of the Body: Medical Knowledge in Britain in the Twentieth Century*.

Just as Foucault found the Panopticon, Armstrong found the Dispensary. Dispensaries were founded towards the end of the 19th century, initially for the screening, diagnosis and treatment of patients with tuberculosis. In this respect they formed an interface between the hospital and the community. But for Armstrong (1983) the dispensary was not only a building which housed a new form of health care; it was 'also a new perceptual structure – a new way of seeing illness which manifested itself in different ways' (p. 8).

The concept of Dispensary (with a capital D to differentiate it from the building) was a new way of construing illness in three respects. Firstly, it involved a new way of organizing health care that radiated into the community. Functioning beyond the walls of the hospital, it acted as a coordinating centre for those who sought out and monitored disease.

Secondly, the medical gaze was diverted from the interior of the physical body to the spaces between bodies. Pathology was not only localized and static, but was found to travel throughout the social body. There was, therefore, a need to focus on contacts, relationships and home visits. Indeed the home became a key site of disciplinary power (Rose, 1985; Nettleton, 1991).

Thirdly, as surveillance extended through the community, the emphasis began to shift from those who were ill to those who were potentially ill. Consequently there was a demise of the binary separation between the normal and abnormal, the ill and the healthy, the mad and the sane. Indeed according to Armstrong (1983), the principal difference between the Panopticon and the Dispensary 'was its denial of the rituals of separation and exclusion that had characterized the exercise of panoptic power' (p. 9).

Thus the Dispensary involved a reorganization of care, a new conceptualization of illness and new forms of observation. These new mechanisms of power which monitored the interactions of people, rather than passive bodies, served to establish a new space. The physical space of the hospital broadened into the social domain of the community.

Like Foucault, Armstrong (1983) draws attention to the inter-relationship between medicine and the human sciences. It is no mere coincidence, he argues, that the Dispensary was founded at the same time that Durkheim was granted the first Chair in sociology. Just as the new organizational structure of medicine was forging the social, so too was the emerging discipline of sociology. Armstrong cites the social survey as the crucial technique in the fabrication of medicine's new object – the person. The survey was an extremely useful tool in this new configuration of medicine, and its refinement facilitated increasingly sophisticated analyses of the community. Indeed, it was the techniques of social research that brought about the reconfiguration of illness from pathological anatomy to the whole person. It was the alliance between the human sciences, both medical and social, that established the subjective patient, the patient's view and, more recently, the 'consumer perspective'.

Illness was no longer the preserve of the medical profession but of the body's own perceptions; the body had to speak, not of some abstract pathological theory of illness, but of immediate feelings. Thus, while the survey became increasingly concerned with the 'objectification' of personal experience through its constant measurement and analysis, it must not be forgotten that those same personal experiences were a fabrication of the creative component of the survey which demanded their visibility. At the very moment as the survey of sickness established its intricate net of surveillance over the whole community it was therefore met by a **rising crescendo of individual expression** (Armstrong, 1983, p. 52, my emphasis).

A REVOLUTION IN MEDICAL CARE

Whilst Dispensary medicine had paved the way for the fabrication of the social domain, it was not until after the Second World War, with the formation of the National Health Service, that the community, and the whole person therein, came to be privileged. From the Foucauldian perspective, these changes are understood in terms of the reformulations of power: 'Comprehensive health care in Britain, from 1948, and contemporary invention and importance of community care are simply manifestations of a new diagram of power which spreads its pervasive gaze throughout a society' (Armstrong, 1983, p. 100).

It would appear, however, that this change in the location of power was not restricted to Britain. Writing in a North American context, Arney and Bergen (1984) argue that a revolution has taken place in medicine which was as important as that described by Foucault as occurring at the end of the 18th century. Just as the first revolution found the docile body, the second revolution found the whole person. By the early 1950s, medicine had invented a new patient through new rules of inquiry. These were no longer organized around a taxonomic logic and anatomical perspectives, prominent in the 19th and early 20th centuries, but were instead based upon a 'systems theoretic logic' and an 'ecological perspective.'

Arney and Bergen (1984) develop their argument by drawing on two images of medicine. The first image is of the anatomy lesson wherein the corpse is dissected to elicit the truth about disease. The second image, which is superimposed upon the first, is that of living persons who are encouraged to speak about their illness so that the truth about their health status can be established.

In this second image, medicine is no longer protecting life from disease. Rather, the doctor's function is to support people so that they will lead healthy lives. Patients are not so much subjected to treatment as: 'managed through experientially optimal courses of events that give people a sense of participation in thrilling adventures' (Arney and Bergen, 1984, p. 163).

It is not, however, simply the medical encounter that has changed. All the other parameters of health care have changed accordingly. For example the health care team extends medicine's reach into the community, and its agents penetrate the school and the home. Lay education aims to ensure that people are monitors of their own health. Contemporary health education, however, does not simply tell people how to behave. The ecological approach requires that they are empowered, and, for this to be possible, it is essential that we understand people's perceptions and motivations. For example Armstrong (1983) notes: 'Health educators who, two decades ago, wrote of the effects of telling people to stop smoking, are now engaged in writing up research which involves asking people for their individual reasons and rationale for smoking' (p. 111).

Similarly, current approaches to alcohol see problem drinking as emerging from the interaction of alcohol, the drinker and the social and physical environment. The drinker is placed in a psychosocial context (Bunton, 1990). Multisectorial programmes are devised which rely on non-segregating and community-based approaches. The drinker participates in his/her treatment by cooperating in such activities as keeping a drinking diary so that he/she may monitor when his/her drinking occurs, and then be proactive in response.

POWER AND PSYCHIATRY

Since the late 1950s, government documents have repeatedly espoused the merits of community as opposed to hospital care for defined client groups such as people with learning difficulties (then the mentally handicapped), the elderly, the physically disabled and the mentally ill (Ham, 1992). Thus far, the emergence of the whole person within the community has been considered in general terms. Now it may be instructive to turn to a more specific example.

When we think about health policies associated with the so-called decanting of hospitals, it is likely that the first area of health care which comes to mind is that of mental health and illness. Three explanations for this change in psychiatric care have been offered: economic, technological and social interest.

Firstly, it has been argued that long-stay in-patient care was expensive and that moving people into the community might have been seen as providing a cheaper alternative. In its Marxist variant, this argument draws attention to the fact that pouring money into large institutions must surely threaten the interests of capital. When money was found to be short, community care solutions looked attractive (Brenner,1973; Dear, Clark and Clark, 1979; Brown, 1988). However, cross-national comparisons have indicated that there is no correlation between financial crises and reduced rates of institutionalized care (Rose, 1986, p. 56). The extent to which community care is a cheaper alternative is also questionable.

The technological explanation points to the contribution of neuroleptic drugs, which appeared on the scene in the 1950s. Pharmaceutical innovations meant that patients were considered able and safe enough (to themselves and others) to live in the community. Such explanations, however, are only relevant to the treatment of mental illness and not to the treatment of people with learning difficulties, the elderly and other groups who were encouraged to stay within the community.

The third, social interests, argument holds that it was the psychiatrists themselves who encouraged the changes in health policy as a means to end their perceived isolation and enhance their status and careers (Scull, 1984; Treacher and Baruch, 1981).

Sociological critiques have drawn on all three arguments, each of which assumes that the rhetoric of humanitarian reforms is used to disguise the true motives for change.

Foucauldian analyses have a different emphasis. They suggest that what the existing critiques have failed to take into account is the transformation of psychiatric knowledge which, in turn, is inextricably interrelated to psychiatric practice (Prior, 1991a, b). In other words, we need to examine the discursive context of psychiatry, that is, what those who speak about psychiatry and mental illness are saying, what they are doing, and, through these activities, what are the objects that they are constructing.

As Prior (1991a) argues: 'each discourse carries with it different objects of focus as well as its own techniques for observing, measuring and organizing such objects' (p. 486). Following a detailed observational study of a long stay psychiatric hospital, Prior concluded that 'the old asylums have been destroyed from within rather than without the walls' (p. 487).

Prior found that the central object within the hospital was the patient's behaviour. Both nursing policy on a psychiatric ward and assessments of patients focused on activities for daily living (ADL). Care plans, for example, were less directed at illness and more at patient behaviours which were observed, assessed and rectified. Behavioural scales, which focused on matters such as the management of money, personal bodily care and clarity of speech, were devised for assessment purposes. Of course other forms of assessment would also be undertaken, but the behavioural ones appeared to be ubiquitous throughout the hospital. Clearly, the best place to assess normal behaviour is within the normal setting. In this respect, institutions are not considered to be particularly conducive and so the community would be a preferable location for those with behavioural problems. This is the nub of Prior's argument. 'My argument is, then, that in choosing behaviour as an object of therapeutic focus psychiatry and psychiatric nursing have lost the rationale they once had for confining themselves within the grounds of a psychiatric hospital. Indeed, the new object of focus has necessitated an extension of professional psychiatric practice into the world "outside"' (Prior, 1991a, p. 487).

Medicine and nursing do not have a monopoly over behaviour. Other kinds of professional involvement become just as legitimate in the management and control of mental illness. Working at the level of behaviour, there is no need to make reference to the underlying psyche or organic malfunctions. Indeed, there has been an expansion of behaviour therapies since the Second World War together with a 'proliferation of sites for the practice of psychiatry' which has involved 'the psychiatrization of new problems and the differentiation of the psychiatric population' (Rose, 1986). There are a whole range of targets, from alcoholics to anorexics to the simply anxious. Psychiatry is now concerned not only with mental illness but with the whole domain of mental health, the potential for which can only be realized within the community. The community, in turn, is constructed by the forms of health care and services that are provided and techniques of social management. 'The community, in the debates over community psychiatry, has a reality which is neither geographical nor that of a network of informal social relationships. It is a social sector, a sector brought into and being marked out by strategies and practices of social management' (Rose, 1986, p. 67).

It is not being assumed that all those involved in psychiatric care are enthusiastic about care in the community. There are the old guard, who prefer the biomedical approach and are sceptical about new forms of care and new types of health professional. However, alternative strategies and techniques are established as a result of debates between the traditionalists and the reformists: 'Hospitals using psychotropic medications, therapeutic communities, feminist self-help groups, social work group homes, community nurses and many other strange bed fellows have combined to chart the domain of mental health and develop technologies for its management' (Rose, 1986, p. 83).

Thus, the critiques of custodial and institutional care have contributed to the reorganization of psychiatry and the creation of new forms of power/knowledge surrounding mental health.

POWER AND HEALTH CARE

Thus far, we have seen how, throughout the 20th century, there has been a shift from hospital to community care which can be understood, from a Foucauldian perspective, in terms of transformation of power from a panoptic to a dispensary regime. More specifically, we have taken the example of psychiatry and seen how there has been a reformulation of psychiatric objects, from the lunatic that manifested an organic malfunction of the brain to the person who manifested abnormal behaviours as a result of his/her social environment.

Foucauldian studies suggest that practitioners in a variety of health care domains have concurrently fabricated comparable medical objects. Psychiatry (Rose, 1985, 1986; Prior, 1991a, b), dentistry (Nettleton, 1992), obstetrics (Arney, 1982) and general medicine (Armstrong, 1983) have fabricated similar objects, namely the biological body of the docile patient, the mind of the unconsciously motivated patient and the social context of the actively thinking and participating patient.

Taking the example of dentistry, Nettleton (1992) has illustrated how, at the turn of the century, the dentist focused only on the physicality of the mouth. By the 1920s, the dentist's gaze had shifted to the mind–mouth complex and, in the postwar years, to the subjective experiencing person. Table 14.1 sets out the techniques and practices that were adopted by dentists, the conceptual spaces within which they were located and the differential objects that dentistry had thereby fabricated.

Table 14.1 A geneaology of dental techniques and dental objects

Dental techniques and practices		*Dental objects*
Population level	*Individual level*	
Epidemiological data: on teeth	Visual inspection	Mouth/teeth
Epidemiological data: personality types and knowledge	Listening/speaking	Mind–mouth complex
Survey data: social circumstances, beliefs, perceptions	Supporting/negotiating	Subjective participating person

The contemporary dental object is the active, thinking person whose personal views and perspectives must be sought if dentistry is to function effectively. The consumer perspective has come to form an integral part of health care.

That there is a compatibility between the findings of studies in these diverse areas of health care adds weight to the thesis that the functioning of power/knowledge transcends professional and disciplinary boundaries. It involves much more than the development of increasingly sophisticated knowledge or political manoeuvrings by those who wish to see a more humane system of health care (Nettleton, 1989, p. 1189).

RISK MANAGEMENT AND CONSUMERISM

Reflecting on contemporary health care, Castel (1991) suggests that we are currently experiencing a further transformation, or revolution, in health care. This change will see:

- the demise of the practitioner–patient relationship;

- a new role for health professionals as health strategists;
- an increasing emphasis on the profiling of populations and the potential marginalization of those groups that do not participate in the postindustrial society.

Castel (1991) conceptualizes these changes in terms of a shift from 'dangerousness' to 'risk'. Hitherto, doctors and psychiatrists, those who have been able to diagnose and prescribe, have treated mental and physical illness. If there was any doubt as to the presence of illness, they were likely to err on the side of caution, so as to prevent manifestation of disease. The patient was thus seen as potentially dangerous.

Currently, the target of medical care is not symptoms but an individual's characteristics that the specialists of prevention policy have constituted as risk factors. The 'clinic of the subject' is being replaced by the 'epidemiological clinic' which is 'a system of multifarious but exactly located expertise which supplants the old doctor–patient relation. This certainly does not mean the end of the doctor, but it does definitely mark a profound transformation in medical practice' (Castel, 1991, p. 282).

We are witnessing the advent of a new mode of surveillance, aided by technological advances, which make the calculus and probabilities of 'systematic predetection' more and more sophisticated. There are two very real consequences of this profound change in medical practice. The first is: 'the separation of diagnosis and treatment, and the transformation of the caring function into an activity of expertise' (Castel, 1991, p. 290).

Practitioners' key function will be to assess their clients and then, on the basis of this assessment, to identify the appropriate route that they should take. Populations are thereby managed on the basis of their profiles, their age, social class, occupation, gender, lifestyles, relationships, where they live, who they live with and so on. It is factors such as these which form their 'risk'.

A second consequence of the change towards risk-oriented practice is that practitioners become subordinate to medical administrators. The mangers of health care are increasingly taking the role of health strategists rather than managing health workers.

> Administration requires an almost complete autonomy because it has virtually absolute control of the new technology. The operative on the ground now becomes a simple auxiliary to a manager who he or she supplies with information derived from the activity of the diagnosis expertise.... These items of information are then stockpiled, processed and distributed along channels completely disconnected from those of professional practice, using in particular the medium of computer data handling (Castel, 1991, p. 293).

Health care is now focusing on needs assessments based on epidemiological and survey data. Strategies are being devised to improve collective health status rather than that of individuals. For example, in response to *The Health of the Nation* (DOH, 1991) the Northern Region Health Authority produced its Regional Health Strategy, called *How do we Create a Healthy North?* (NRHA, 1992). This strategy identified targets in the form of the collective reduction of risk factors and the development of a network of effective health care and social services. 'The strategy will be successful if it finds ways to modify risk factors on a scale and to help adopt and sustain choices in their lives which are supportive to health rather than harmful and injurious.'

The document was consultative, and its objective was to incorporate the consumer's perspective. Thus the consumer's voice now forms a central strand in health care and health care policy. The political debate about the extent to which the consumer is really listened to will, of course, continue. This is crucial because, as we have seen, it is debates between the opposing factions of those involved in health care that help to keep the issues alive. Such debates are especially important in those areas in which health services users are being encouraged by professional groups to stay within the hospital (see the discussion of midwifery in Chapter 5).

Today, health care increasingly takes place within the context of the community and 'hospitals at home'. The role of the hospital is diminishing, and more care for patients with conditions such as diabetes, AIDS, asthma, stroke, renal failure and other chronic conditions is taking place at home. Just as the appearance of the teaching hospitals fabricated pathological anatomy, so the emphasis on care in the community has realized the participating patient.

It is no coincidence that a report has recommended that the number of teaching hospitals in London needs to be reduced and that a greater proportion of medical education should take place in the community (Tomlinson, 1992). This is not simply an outcome of internal markets which has led to a decline in demand for London's expensive acute services. It is also an effect of a reconfiguration of disciplinary power. Patients and carers will be assessed by a range of professionals and in a range of settings. The community comprises a whole network of hospitals and homes, day centres, rehabilitation units, private residential homes, educational centres and so on. Community health services form alliances with other agencies and patients who, on the basis of their profiles, will be involved in initiating and managing the individual's trajectory.

References

Aarvold, J. (1989) Mothers speak out on antenatal care. *Maternity Care in Action*, October, 8.

Abberley, P. (1987) The concept of oppression and the development of a social theory of disability. *Disability, Handicap and Society*, **2**, 5–19.

Ackerknecht, E.H. (1967) *Medicine at the Paris Hospital 1794–1848*, Johns Hopkins Press, Baltimore, MD.

Amoss, A., Jones, L. and Martin, C. (1988) *A Report on a Survey of Users' Opinions. Commissioned by The Maternity Service Group of Edinburgh Local Health Council*, Department of Community Medicine, University of Edinburgh, Edinburgh.

Appleby, J., Smith, P., Ranade, W. *et al.* (1994) Monitoring managed competition, in *Evaluating the NHS Reforms*, (eds R. Robinson and J. Le Grand), King's Fund, London.

Armstrong, D. (1983) *Political Anatomy of the Body: Medical Knowledge in Britain in the Twentieth Century*, Cambridge University Press, Cambridge.

Armstrong, D. (1990) Use of the genealogical method in the exploration of chronic illness: a research note. *Social Science and Medicine*, **30**, 1225–1227.

Arney, W.R. (1982) *Power and the Profession of Obstetrics*, University of Chicago Press, London.

Arney, W.R. and Bergen, B.J. (1984) *Medicine and the Management of Living: Taming the Last Great Beast*, University of Chicago Press, London.

Artells, J. (1988) Effectiveness and decision making in health planning context: the case of outpatient antenatal care, in *The Economics of Health Care*, (eds A. McGuire, J. Henderson and G. Mooney), Routledge & Kegan Paul, London.

Ashton, J. and Seymour, H. (1988) *The New Public Health*, Open University Press, Milton Keynes.

Association of Community Health Councils for England and Wales (1987) *Antenatal Care: Still Waiting for Action. Health News Briefing*, ACHCEW, London.

Astrom, S., Nilsson, M., Norberg, A. *et al.* (1991) Staff burnout in dementia care – relations to empathy and attitudes. *International Journal of Nursing Studies*, **28**, 65–75.

Audit Commission (1986) *Making a Reality of Community Care*, HMSO, London.

Badger, F., Evers, H. and Cameron, E. (1989) *The Community Care Project: Community Service Provision and Clients with Dementia*, Report no. 29, Department of Social Medicine, University of Birmingham, Birmingham.

Baker, F. and Intagliata, J. (1982) Quality of life: some measurement requirements, *Evaluation and Programme Planning*, **5**, 69–79.

Baldwin, S. (1993) *The Myth of Community Care: An Alternative Neighbourhood Model of Care*, Chapman & Hall, London.

Banks, C., Maloney, E. and Willcock, H.D. (1975) Public attitudes to crime and the penal system. *British Journal of Criminology*, **15**, 228–240.

Barclay, L. (1986) Midwifery: a case of misleading packaging? *Australian Journal of Advanced Nursing*, **3**, 21–26.

Bartlett, W. and Harrison, L. (1993) Quasi-markets and the national health service reforms, in *Quasi-Markets and Social Policy*, (eds J. Le Grand and W. Bartlett), Macmillan, Basingstoke.

Basch, C.E. (1987) Focus group interview: an under-utilized research technique for improving theory and practice in health education. *Health Education Quarterly*, **14**, 411–448.

Beck, U. (1992) *Risk Society: Towards a New Modernity*, Sage Publications, London.

Becker, M.H. (1974) *The Health Belief Model and Personal Health Behavior*, Charles B. Slack, Thorofare, NJ.

Beedham, H. and Wilson-Barnett, J. (1991) *Evaluation of Services for People with HIV/AIDS: A Nursing Study*, University of London, London.

Bell, R., Gibbons, S. and Pinchen, I. (1987) *Action Research with Informal Carers of Elderly People*, Health Education Services, Cambridge.

Belson, W.A. (1981) *The Design and Understanding of Survey Questions*, Gower, Aldershot.

Benjamin, A. (1989) Perspectives on a continuum of care for persons with HIV illnesses, in *New Perspectives on HIV-Related Illnesses: Progress in Health Services Research*, (ed. W.N. LeVee), National Center for Health Services Research and Health Care Technology Assessment, Rockville, MD.

Benyon, J. (1993) *Crime, Order and Policing: Studies in Crime, Order and Policing*, Occasional Paper No 1, Centre for the Study of Public Order, University of Leicester, Leicester.

Block, R. (1980) Factors related to maternal overprotection of the mentally retarded adult. School of Human Behaviour, United States International University. Dissertation.

Blumer, H. (1969) *Symbolic Interactionism*, Prentice Hall, Englewood Cliffs, NJ.

Bond, J. (1992) The politics of caregiving: the professionalisation of informal care. *Ageing and Society*, **12**, 5–21.

Bond, J. and Coleman, P. (1990) Ageing into the twenty-first century, in *Ageing in Society: An Introduction to Social Gerontology*,(eds J. Bond and P. Coleman), Sage Publications, London.

Bond, T. (1990) *HIV Counselling Report on National Survey and Consultation 1990*, British Association for Counselling/Department of Health Joint Project, London.

Bowling, A., Jacobson, B. and Southgate, L. (1993) Health service priorities: explorations in consultation of the public and health professionals on priority setting in an inner London health district. *Social Science and Medicine*, **7**, 851–857.

Boyd, C. and Sellers, L. (1982) *The British Way of Birth*, Pan, London.

Bradshaw, J. (1972) The concept of social need. *New Society*, **30**, 640–643.

Brenner, M.H. (1973) *Mental Illness and the Economy*, Harvard University Press, Cambridge, MA.

Brewer, C. (1986) Patterns of compliance and evasion in treatment programmes which include supervised disulfiram. *Alcohol and Alcoholism*, **21**, 385–388.

Brody, E.M. and Brody, S.J. (1974) Decade of decision for the elderly. *Social Work*, **19**, 544–554.

Brotherston, J. (1976) Inequality: is it inevitable?, in *Equalities and Inequalities in Health*, (eds C.O. Carter and J. Peel), Academic Press, London.

Brown, P. (1988) Recent trends in the political economy of mental health, in *Location and Stigma: Perspectives on Mental Health and Mental Health Care*, (eds C.J. Smith and J.A. Giggs), Unwin Hyman, London.

Bryman, A. (1988) *Quantity and Quality in Social Research*, Unwin Hyman, London.

Bulmer, M. (1979) *Censuses, Surveys and Privacy*, Macmillan, Basingstoke.

Bulmer, M. (1982) *The Uses of Social Research: Social Investigation in Public Policy-Making*, Allen & Unwin, London.

Bunton, R. (1990) Regulating our favourite drug, in *New Directions in the Sociology of Health*, (eds P. Abbott and G. Payne), Falmer, London.

Burgess, A. (1993) The problem of waiting for years: a qualitative study of people waiting for hip replacement therapy. Institute of Health Sciences, University of Northumbria, Newcastle-upon-Tyne, Postgraduate Diploma Thesis.

Burgess, R.G. (1984) *In the Field: An Introduction to Field Research*, Unwin Hyman, London.

Buswell, C. (1980) Mothers' perceptions of professionals in child health care. Unpublished paper given at Community Paediatric Research Club meeting, December.

Butler, A. and Pritchard, C. (1983) *Social Work and Mental Illness*, Macmillan, Basingstoke.

Butler J. (1994) Origins and early developments, in *Evaluating the NHS Reforms*, (eds R. Robinson and J. Le Grand), King's Fund, London.

Byrne, G.S.M. (1992) The Accident and Emergency Department: nurses' priorities and patients' anxieties. University of Northumbria, PhD Thesis.

Calnan, M. (1984) The functions of the hospital emergency department: a study of patient demand. *Journal of Emergency Medicine*, **2**, 57–63.

Calnan, M. (1988) Lay evaluation of medicine and medical practice: report of a pilot study. *International Journal of Health Services*, **18**, 311–322.

Campbell, R. and Macfarlane, A. (1987) *Where to be Born: The Debate and the Evidence*, National Perinatal Epidemiology Unit, Radcliffe Infirmary, Oxford.

Carers' National Association (1994) *Community Care: Just a Fairy Tale?*, Carers' National Association, London.

Carpenter, M. (1994) *Normality is Hard Work: Trade Unionism and the Politics of Community Care*, Lawrence and Wishart/Unison, London.

Carr, J. (1975) *Young Children with Down's Syndrome*, Butterworth, London.

Carr-Hill , R.A. (1989) Assumptions of the QALY Procedure. *Social Science and Medicine*, **29**, 469–477.

Castel, R. (1991) From dangerousness to risk, in *The Foucault Effect: Studies in Governmentality*, (eds G. Burchell, C. Gordon and P. Miller), Harvester Wheatsheaf, Brighton.

Catalan, J., Marsack, P., Hawton, K.E. *et al.* (1980) Comparison of doctors and nurses in the assessment of deliberate self-poisoning patients. *Psychological Medicine*, **10**, 483–491.

Cattermole, M., Jahoda, A. and Markova, I. (1987) Training for independent living in mental hospitals and ATCs. University of St Andrews, Mimeograph.

Central Statistics Office (1986) *Social Trends 16*, HMSO, London.

Challis, D., Chessum, R., Chesterman, J. *et al.* (1987) Community care for the frail elderly: an urban experiment. *British Journal of Social Work*, **18**, 13–41.

Chenoweth, B. and Spencer, B. (1986) Dementia: the experience of family care-givers. *Gerontologist*, **26**, 267–272.

Cicourel, A.V. (1973) *Cognitive Sociology*, Penguin, Harmondsworth.

Clark, J. (1973) *A Family Visitor*, Royal College of Nursing, London.

Clark, J. (1981) *What Do Health Visitors Do?: A Review of the Research 1960–1980*, Royal College of Nursing, London.

Clarke, C.L. (1989) The interrelationships between the dementing elderly, their informal and formal carers, and the implications for nursing provision. Institute of Health Sciences, University of Northumbria, MSc Thesis.

Clarke, C.L., Heyman, B., Pearson, P. and Watson, D.W. (1993) Formal carers: attitudes to working with the dementing elderly and their informal carers. *Health and Social Care*, 1, 227–238.

Clarke, C.L. and Watson, D. (1991) Informal carers of the dementing elderly: a study of relationships. *Nursing Practice*, 4, 17–21.

Clarke, K. (1982) Patient health teaching needs. *Journal of Emergency Nursing*, 8, 298–303.

Cliff, K. and Wood, T (1986a) Accident and emergency departments: why people attend with minor injuries and ailments. *Public Health*, 100, 15–29.

Cliff, K. and Wood, T. (1986b) Accident and emergency services: the ambulant patient. *Hospital and Health Services Review*, 82, 74–77.

Clulow, C.F. (1982) *To Have and To Hold: Marriage, the First Baby and Preparing Couples for Parenthood*, Aberdeen University Press, Aberdeen.

Cohen, A.P. (1985) *The Symbolic Construction of Community*, Ellis Horwood, Chichester.

Collins, J. (1993) *The Resettlement Game: Policy and Procrastination in the Closure of Mental Handicap Hospitals*, Values into Action, London.

Cook, T.D. and Campbell, D.T. (1979) *Quasi-Experimentation: Design and Analysis Issues for Field Settings*, Rand McNally, Chicago, IL.

Cormack, D. (1992) *The Research Process in Nursing*, Blackwell, Oxford.

Cornwell, J. (1984) *Hard Earned Lives: Accounts of Health and Illness from East London*, Tavistock Publications, London.

Council for the Education and Training of Health Visitors (1977) *An Investigation into the Principles of Health Visiting*, CETHV, London.

Counsel and Care (1993) *People Not Parcels: A Discussion Document to Explore the Issues Surrounding the use of Electronic Tagging on Older People in Residential Care and Nursing Homes*, Counsel and Care, London.

Counsel and Care (1994) *More Power to Our Elders*, Counsel and Care, London.

Cowley, S. (1991) A symbolic awareness context identified through a grounded theory study of health visiting. *Journal of Advanced Nursing*, 16, 648–656.

Critchfield, G.C. and Eddy, D.M. (1987) A confidence profile analysis of disulfiram in the treatment of chronic alcoholism. *Medical Care*, 25, 566–575.

Cunningham, D. (1989a) Key issues for planning, in *AIDS: Models of Care*, (eds M. Bould and G. Peacock), King's Fund/London Boroughs Training Committee, London.

Daley, M. (1993) *Outercourse*, Women's Press, London.

Dalley, G. (1988) *Ideologies of Caring: Rethinking Community and Collectivism*, Macmillan, Basingstoke.

Dalley, G. (1993) Professional ideology or organizational tribalism? The health service–social work divide, in *Health and Welfare Practice*, (eds J. Walmsley, J. Reynolds, P. Shakespeare and R. Woolfe), Sage Publications/Open University, London.

Danis, D. (1984) Fear in emergency department patients. *Journal of Emergency Nursing*, 10, 151–155.

Davey Smith, G., Bartley, M. and Blane, D. (1990) The Black Report on inequalities in health: 10 years on. *British Medical Journal*, 301, 373–377.

Davies, J. (1982) Dangers in the policy against home confinements. *Science and Public Policy*, 9, 286–291.

Davison, A.G., Hildrey, A.C. and Floyer, M.A. (1983) Use and misuse of an accident and emergency service in the east end of London. *Journal of the Royal Society of Medicine*, 76, 37–40.

Day, G. and Murdoch, J. (1993) Locality and community: coming to terms with place. *Sociological Review*, 41, 82–111.

Dear, M., Clark, G. and Clark, S. (1979) Economic cycles and mental health care policy: an examination of the macro-context for social service planning. *Social Science and Medicine*, **13c**, 43–53.

Delbecq, A.L. and Van der Ven, A.H. (1971) A group process model for problem identification and programme planning. *Journal of Applied Behavioural Science*, **7**, 466–492.

Dey, I. (1993) *Qualitative Data Analysis: A User-Friendly Guide for Social Scientists*, Routledge, London.

DHSS (1981) Growing Older, *Cmnd. 8173*, HMSO, London.

Dingwall, R. (1977) *The Social Organisation of Health Visitor Training*, Croom Helm, London.

Division of Obstetrics and Gynaecology (1993) *Response to Consultation Paper on the Provision of Maternity Services: 6. Other Developments*, Division of Obstetrics and Gynaecology, Newcastle-upon-Tyne

Dixon, J. and Welch, H.G. (1991) Priority setting: lessons from Oregon. *Lancet*, **337**, 891–894.

Dixon, P.N. and Morris, A.F. (1971) Casual attendances at an accident and emergency department and health centre. *British Medical Journal*, **4**, 214–216.

DOH (1989) *Caring for People: Community Care in the Next Decade and Beyond*, HMSO, London.

DOH (1990) *Contracts for Health Services: Operational Principles*, HMSO, London.

DOH (1991) *The Health of the Nation*, HMSO, London.

DOH (1993) *Changing Childbirth, Part 1: Report of the Expert Maternity Group, Chair Baroness Cumberledge*, HMSO, London

Donaldson, C., Clark, K., Gregson, B. et al. (1988) *Evaluation of a Family Support Unit for Elderly Mentally Infirm People and their Carers*, Report no. 34, Health Care Research Unit, University of Newcastle upon Tyne.

Donavon, D.M. and Marlatt, G.A. (1988) *Assessment of Addictive Behaviours*, Guilford Press, New York.

Drane, J.W. (1991) Imputing nonresponses to mail-back questionnaires. *American Journal of Epidemiology*, **134**, 908–912.

Driscoll, P.A., Vincent, C. and Wilkinson, M. (1987) The use and misuse of the accident and emergency department. *Accident and Emergency Medicine*, **4**, 77–82.

Dunnell, K. and Dobbs, J. (1982) *Nurses Working in the Community*, Office of Population Censuses and Surveys, Social Survey Division, HMSO, London.

Eaves, J.D. (1986) Extended role activities, triage and the management of the required total care of patients with minor injuries/complaints: a survey of accident and emergency nurses' practices and attitudes. University of Manchester, MSc Thesis.

Eayrs, C.B., Ellis, N. and Jones, S.P. (1993) Which label? An investigation into the effects of terminology on public perceptions of and attitudes towards people with learning difficulties. *Handicap, Disability and Society*, **8**, 111–128.

Egan, G. (1986) *The Skilled Helper*, Brooks/Cole, Pacific Grove, CA.

Elbourne, D., Richardson, M., Chalmers, I. et al. (1987) The Newbury Maternity Care Study: a randomised controlled trial to assess a policy of women holding their own obstetric records. *British Journal of Obstetrics and Gynaecology*, **94**, 612–619.

Eley, R. and Middleton, L. (1983) Square pegs, round holes. The appropriateness of providing care for old people in residential settings. *Health Trends*, **15**, 68–70.

Enkin, M. and Chalmers, I. (1982) *Effectiveness and Satisfaction in Antenatal Care*, Heinemann, London.

Evans, F. (1987) *The Newcastle Community Midwifery Care Project: An Evaluation Report*, Newcastle Health Authority, Newcastle-upon-Tyne.

Evans, G. and Murcott, A. (1990) Community care: relationships and control. *Disability, Handicap and Society*, **5**, 123–135.

Fagerhaugh, S.Y. (1986) Analysing data for basic social processes, in *From Practice to Grounded Theory*, (eds W.C. Chenitz and J.M. Swanson), Addison-Wesley, California.

Faris, R.E. and Dunham, H.W. (1939) *Mental Disorders in Urban Areas*, University of Chicago Press, Chicago, IL.

Felce, D., Taylor, D. and Wright, K. (1992) *People with Learning Disabilities*, DHA Project: Research Programme: Epidemiologically Based Needs Assessment, Report 12, NHSME, London.

Field, S., Draper, J., Kerr, M. & Hare, M. (1982) A consumer view of the health visiting service. *Health Visitor*, **57**, 273–275.

Finch, J. (1984) 'It's great to have someone to talk to': the ethics and politics of interviewing women, in *Social Researching: Politics, Problems, Practice*, (eds C. Bell and H. Roberts), Routledge & Kegan Paul, London.

Fitzpatrick, R. and Hopkins, A. (1983) Problems in the conceptual framework of patient satisfaction research: an empirical exploration. *Sociology of Health and Illness*, **5**, 297–311.

Flint, C. and Poulengeris, P. (1987) *The 'Know your Midwife' Report*, 49 Peckarmans Wood, London SE26 6RZ.

Flynn, M. and Saleem, J. (1986) Adults who are mentally handicapped and living with their parents: satisfaction and perceptions regarding their lives and circumstances. *Journal of Mental Deficiency*, **30**, 379–387.

Foucault, M. (1976) *The Birth of the Clinic: An Archaeology of Medical Perception*, Tavistock Publications, London.

Foucault, M. (1979) *Discipline and Punish: The Birth of the Prison*, Penguin Books, London.

Fox, J.G. and Storms, D.M. (1981) A different approach to sociodemographic predictors of satisfaction with health care. *Social Science and Medicine*, **15A**, 557–564.

Franklin, J., Simmons, J., Soloviitz, B. *et al.* (1986) Assessing quality of life of the mentally ill. *Evaluation and the Health Professions*, **9**, 376–388.

Friedman, M. (1962) *Capitalism and Freedom*, University of Chicago Press, Chicago, IL.

Friedson, E. (1961) *Patients' View of Medical Practice*, Russell Sage, New York.

Furnham, A. (1983) Mental health and employment status: a preliminary study. *British Journal of Guidance and Counselling*, **11**, 197–201.

Gabe, J. and Bury, M. (1991) Tranquillisers and health care in crisis. *Social Science and Medicine*, **32**, 449–454.

Garcia, J., Kilpatrick, R. and Richards, M. (1990) *The Politics of Maternity Care*, Clarendon Press, Oxford.

Gatherer, A., Parfit, J., Porter, E. and Vessey, M. (1980) *Is Health Education Effective?*, Health Education Council Monograph, Health Education Council, London.

Gibson, H. (1977) Rules, routines and records: the work of an Accident and Emergency Department. University of Aberdeen, PhD Thesis.

Giddens, A. (1991) *Modernity and Self-Identity: Self and Society in the Late Modern Age*, Polity, Oxford.

Gilhooly, M.L.M. (1984) The impact of care-giving on caregivers: factors associated with the psychological well-being of people supporting a dementing relative in the community, *British Journal of Medical Psychology*, **57**, 35–44.

Glaser, B.G and Strauss, A.L. (1967) *The Discovery of Grounded Theory Strategies for Qualitative Research*, Aldine Press, Chicago, IL.

Goffman, E. (1961) *Asylums: Essays on the Social Situations of Mental Patients and Other Patients*, Anchor, New York.

Goffman, E. (1971) *Relations in Public: Microstudies of the Public Order*, Harper, New York.

Goldberg, D.P. and Hillier, V.F. (1979) A scaled version of the General Health Questionnaire. *Psychological Medicine*, **9**, 139–145.

Goldsmith, J. and Thomas, N.E. (1974) Crimes against the elderly: a continuing national crisis. *Aging*, **236**, 10–13.

Goodwin, S (1982) *Whither Health Visiting?*, Health Visitors Association, London.

Goodwin, S. (1990) *Community Care and the Future of Mental Health Service Provision*, Avebury, Aldershot.

Graham, H. (1979) Women's attitudes to the child health services. *Health Visitor*, **52**, 175–178.

Graham, H. (1984) Surveying through stories, in *Social Researching: Politics, Problems, Practice*, (eds C. Bell and H. Roberts), Routledge & Kegan Paul, London.

Graham, H. and Oakley, A. (1981) Competing ideologies of reproduction, in *Women, Health and Reproduction*, (ed. H. Roberts), Routledge & Kegan Paul, London.

Green, J. and Dale, J. (1992) Primary care in accident and emergency and general practice: a comparison. *Social Science and Medicine*, **35**, 987–995.

Green, J., Dale, J. and Glucksman, E. (1991) Half the aggro. *Health Service Journal*, **101**, 25.

Griffiths, R. (Chairman) (1983) *NHS Management Inquiry (Recommendations to the Secretary of State for Social Services, October 1983)*, DHSS, London.

Griffiths, R. (1988a) Does the public serve? The consumer dimension. *Public Administration*, **66**, 195–204.

Griffiths, R. (1988b) *Community Care: Agendas for Action*, HMSO, London.

Grimshaw, J. (1989) The South London HIV Centre: the Landmark, in *AIDS: Models of Care*, (eds M. Bould and G. Peacock), King's Fund/London Boroughs Training Committee, London.

Gulbenkian Foundation (1968) *Community Work and Social Change*, Longman, Harlow.

Habermas, J. (1984) *The Theory of Communicative Action, Volume One: Reason and the Rationalisation of Society*, Heinemann, London.

Hald, J. and Jacobsen, E. (1948) A drug sensitising the organism to ethyl alcohol. *Lancet*, **255**, 1001.

Haley, W.E., Brown, E.G., Brown, S.L. *et al.* (1987) Psychological, social and health consequences of caring for a relative with senile dementia. *Journal of the American Geriatrics Society*, **35**, 405–411.

Ham, C. (1992) *Health Policy in Britain: The Politics and Organisation of the National Health Service*, Macmillan, Basingstoke.

Handyside, E.C. (1989) 'Mind's eye': clients' perceptions of community mental health care. Institute of Health Sciences, University of Northumbria, MSc Thesis.

Handyside, E.C. and Heyman, R. (1990) Community mental health care: clients' perceptions of services and an evaluation of a voluntary agency support scheme. *International Journal of Social Psychiatry*, **36**, 280–290.

Hanson, B.S. and Ostergren, P.O. (1987) Different social network and social support characteristics, nervous problems and insomnia: theoretical and methodological aspects of some results from the population study 'Men Born in 1914', Malmo, Sweden. *Social Science and Medicine*, **25**, 849–859.

Hare, D. (1972) *The Cultural Warping of Childbirth*, International Childbirth Association, Seattle, WA.

Harré, R. and Secord, P.F. (1972) *The Explanation of Social Behaviour*, Blackwell, Oxford.

Harrington, B., White, M., Foy, C. *et al.* (1993) *The Newcastle Health and Lifestyle Survey 1991: Health and Lifestyles in Newcastle*, University of Newcastle, Newcastle-upon-Tyne.

Hatch, S. and Kickbusch, I. (eds) (1983) *Self Help and Health in Europe*, WHO Regional Office for Europe, Copenhagen.

Health Advisory Service (1982) *Northern Region Report*, HMSO, London.

Health Visitors Association (1981) *Health Visiting in the Eighties*, HVA, London.

Heather, N. and Robertson, I. (1985) *Problem Drinking: The New Approach*, Pelican, Harmondsworth.

Hedges, A. (1985) Group interviewing, in *Applied Qualitative Research*, (ed. R. Walker), Gower, Aldershot.

Heumann, L. and Boldy, D. (1982) *Housing for the Elderly*, Croom Helm, London.

Heyman, B. and Huckle, S. (1993a) 'Normal' life in a hazardous world. How adults with moderate learning difficulties cope with risks and dangers. *Disability, Handicap and Society*, **8**, 143–160.

Heyman, B. and Huckle, S. (1993b) Not worth the risk? Attitudes of adults with learning difficulties and their informal and formal carers to the hazards of everyday life. *Social Science and Medicine*, **12**, 1557–1564.

Hicks, C. (1992) Research in midwifery: are midwives their own worst enemy? *Midwifery*, **8**, 12–18.

HMSO (1993) *Households Below Average Income 1979–1990/91*, HMSO, London.

HMSO (1994) *A Prescription for Improvement*, HMSO, London.

Hodgson, J. (1992) First flush of success for diagnosing diabetes. *New Scientist*, **1852/1853**, 20.

Hodnett, E.D. (1989) Personal control and the birth environment: comparisons between home and hospital settings. *Journal of Environmental Psychology*, **9**, 207–216.

Hofman, A., Rocca,W.A., Brayne, C. *et al.* (1991) The prevalence of dementia in Europe: a collaborative study of 1980–1990 findings. *International Journal of Epidemiology*, **20**, 736–748.

Horrocks, P. (1985) Performance indicators. *Health and Social Service Journal*, **94**, 803.

House of Commons Health Committee (1992) *Maternity Services, Chair Nicholas Winterton MP*, HMSO, London.

House of Commons Health Committee (1994) *Better Off in the Community? The Care of People Who are Seriously Mentally Ill*, HMSO, London.

House of Commons Social Services Committee (1980) *Perinatal and Neonatal Mortality: Second Report from the Social Services Committee*, HMSO, London.

Howarth, O. (1989) *Textile Voices: Mill Life this Century*, Bradford Heritage Recording Unit, Bradford.

Hubley, J.H. (1980) Community development and health education. *Journal of the Institute of Health Education*, **18**, 113–120.

Hughes, D. (1989) Paper and people: the work of the casualty reception clerk. *Sociology of Health and Illness*, **11**, 382–407.

Hughes, E.C. (1960) Introduction: the place of fieldwork in social science, in *Field Work: An Introduction to the Social Sciences*, (ed. B. Junker), University of Chicago Press, Chicago, IL.

Hugman, R. (1991) *Power in Caring Professions*, Macmillan, Basingstoke.

Hulley, S.B., Newman, T.B., Grady, D. *et al.* (1993) Should we be measuring blood cholesterol levels in young adults? *Journal of the American Medical Association,* **269**, 1416–1419.

Hunter, M. (1994) The impact of the NHS reforms on community care, in *Caring for People in the Community: The New Welfare,* (ed. M. Titterton), Jessica Kingsley, London.

Inch, S. (1981) *Birthrights,* Hutchinson, London.

Irving, M. (1988) *The Management of Patients with Major Injuries: Report of the Working Party of the Royal College of Surgeons,* Royal College of Surgeons, London.

Jacoby, A. (1990) Possible factors affecting response to postal questionnaires: findings from a study of general practitioner services. *Journal of Public Health Medicine,* **12**, 131–135.

Jacoby, A. and Cartwright, A. (1990) Finding out about the views and experiences of maternity service users, in *The Politics of Maternity Care,* (eds J. Garcia, R. Kilpatrick and M. Richards), Clarendon Press, Oxford.

James, N. (1992) Care = organisation + physical labour + emotional labour. *Sociology of Health and Illness,* **14**, 488–509.

Jeffrey, R. (1979) Normal rubbish: deviant patients in casualty departments. *Sociology of Health and Illness,* **1**, 90–107.

Johnson, T.J. (1972) *Professions and Power,* Macmillan, London.

Jones, D., Lester, C. and West, R. (1994) Monitoring changes in health services for older people, in *Evaluating the NHS Reforms,* (eds R. Robinson and J. Le Grand), King's Fund, London.

Jowitt, M. (1993) *Childbirth Unmasked,* Peter Wooller, Walford Lodge, Walford, Shropshire.

Kaplan, A. (1964) *The Conduct of Inquiry,* Chandler, San Francisco, CA.

Katz, A. and Bender, E.I. (eds) (1976) *The Strength In Us: Self Help Groups in the Modern World,* Franklin Watts, New York.

Katz-Rothman, B. (1982) *In Labour: Woman and Power in the Birthplace,* Junction Books, London.

Kelly, G.A. (1955) *The Psychology of Personal Constructs: 1 – A Theory of Personality,* Norton, New York (reprinted by Routledge, London, 1991).

Kelly, M. and May, D. (1982) Good and bad patients: a review of the literature and a theoretical critique. *Journal of Advanced Nursing,* **7**, 147–156.

Kennedy, I. (1983) Showbiz and the doctors: why *Panorama* was wrong. *Sunday Times,* **13 November.**

Kilian, A. (1988) Conscientisation: an empowering, nonformal education approach to community health workers. *Community Development Journal,* **23**, 117–123.

King, M. (1989) Prejudice and AIDS: the views and experiences of people with HIV Infection. *AIDS Care,* **1**, 137–143.

Kingsley, S. and Douglas, R. (1991) Developing service strategies: the transition to community care, in *Managing Community Health Services,* (ed. A. McNaught), Chapman & Hall, London.

Kirk, J. and Miller, M.L. (1986) *Reliability and Validity in Qualitative Research,* Sage Publications, Beverly Hills, CA.

Kirkham, M. (1989) Midwives and information-giving during labour, in *Midwives Research and Childbirth,* vol. 1, (eds S. Robinson and A.M. Thomson), Chapman & Hall, London.

Kitzinger, J. (1994) The methodology of focus groups: the importance of interaction between research participants. *Sociology of Health and Illness,* **16**, 103–121.

Kitzinger, S. (1978) *The Experience of Childbirth,* Penguin, Harmondsworth.

Krueger, R.A. (1988) *Focus Groups: A Practical Guide for Applied Research*, Sage Publications, Beverly Hills, CA.

Laing, R.D., Phillipdon, H. and Lee, A.R. (1966) *Interpersonal Perception: A Theory and a Method of Research*, Tavistock Publications, London.

Laslett, B. and Rapoport, R. (1975) Collaborative interviewing and interactive research. *Journal of Marriage and the Family*, **37**, 968–977.

Layzell, S. and McCarthy, M. (1992) Community based health services for people with HIV/AIDS: a review from a health service perspective. *AIDS Care*, **4**, 203–215.

Le Grand, J. and Bartlett, W. (1993) *Quasi-Markets and Social Policy*, Macmillan, Basingstoke.

L'État de la France (1993) Editions La Decoverte, Paris.

Lewis, B.R. and Bradbury, Y. (1982) The role of the nursing profession in hospital accident and emergency departments. *Journal of Advanced Nursing*, **7**, 211–221.

Lewis, C. (1986) *Becoming a Father*, Open University Press, Milton Keynes.

Liggins, K. (1993) Inappropriate attendance at accident and emergency departments: a literature review. *Journal of Advanced Nursing*, **18**, 1141–1145.

Link, B.G. (1987) Understanding labelling effects in the area of mental disorders: an assessment of the effects of expectations and rejection. *American Sociological Review*, **52**, 96–112.

Lomas, P. (1964) Childbirth rituals. *New Society*, **4**, 118.

Lovell, A., Zander, L., James, C. *et al.* (1986) *St. Thomas' Maternity Case Notes Study: Why Not Give Women Their Own Case Notes?* Cicely Northcote Trust, London.

Lowe, R. (1993) *The Welfare State in Britain Since 1945*, Macmillan, Basingstoke.

Luker, K. (1982) *Evaluating Health Visiting Practice*, Royal College of Nursing, London.

Lukes, S. (1974) *Power: A Radical View*, Macmillan, London.

Lynott, R.J. (1983) Alzheimer's disease and institutionalisation. *Journal of Family Issues*, **4**, 559–574.

McCann, K. (1990) Care in the community and by the community. *AIDS Care*, **2**, 421–424.

McCann, K. (1991) The work of a specialist AIDS home support team: the views and experiences of patients using the service. *Journal of Advanced Nursing*, **16**, 832–836.

McCann, K. and Wadsworth, E. (1992) The role of informal carers in supporting gay men who have HIV related illnesses: what do they do and what are their needs? *AIDS Care*, **4**, 25–33.

McCool, W.F. and McCool, S.J. (1989) Feminism and nurse midwifery: historical overview and current issues. *Journal of Nurse Midwifery*, **34**, 323–334.

Macdonald, G. and Smith, C. (1990) Complacency, risk perception and the problem of HIV education. *AIDS Care*, **2**, 63–68.

McEwan, L. (1989) Community care and accommodation, in *AIDS: Models of Care*, (eds M. Bould and G. Peacock), King's Fund/London Boroughs Training Committee, London.

Machin, T.A. (1993) Back-up, breathing space and commitment to abstinence: an exploratory study of the meaning and influence of disulfiram therapy from a client perspective. Institute of Health Sciences, University of Northumbria, MSc Thesis.

McIver, S. (1992) Measurement of patient opinions, in Health Care in Europe After 1992, (eds H.E.G.M. Hermans, A.F. Casparie and J.H.P. Paelinck), Erasmus University Rotterdam/Dartmouth, Aldershot, UK.

McIver, S. (1993) *Obtaining the Views of Users of Primary and Community Health Care Services*, King's Fund, London.

McKee, I. (1984) Community antenatal care: the Sighthill Community Clinic, in *Pregnancy Care for the 1980s*, (eds L. Zander and G. Chamberlain), Macmillan, London.

McKeown, K., Whitelaw, S., Hambleton, D. and Green, F. (1994) Setting priorities – science art or politics?, in *Setting Priorities in Health Care*, (ed. M. Malek), John Wiley, Chichester.

MacLeod, E. and Mein, P. (1987) The nursing care team: a task force approach, in *Preventative Care of the Elderly: A Review of Current Developments*, (eds R.C. Taylor and E.G. Buckley), Occasional Paper 35, Royal College of General Practitioners,London.

Mangen, S.P. and Griffith, J.H. (1982) Patient satisfaction with community psychiatric nursing: a prospective controlled study. *Journal of Advanced Nursing*, **7**, 477–482.

Market Research Society (1979) Qualitative research: a summary of the concepts involved. *Journal of the Market Research Society*, **21**, 107–124.

Marks, D.F. (1994) Psychology's role in *The Health of the Nation*, *Psychologist*, **7**, 119–121.

Marsh C. (1982) *The Survey Method: The Contribution of Surveys to Sociological Explanation*, Allen & Unwin, London.

Mawby, R.I. (1982) Crime and the elderly: a review of British and American research. *Current Psychological Reviews*, **2**, 301–310.

Mayall, B. (1986) *Keeping Children Healthy*, Allen & Unwin, London.

Mayall, B. and Grossmith, C. (1985) The health visitor and the provision of services. *Health Visitor*, **58**, 349–352.

Maynard, A. (1992) *Is it Helpful to Measure the Social Costs of Alcohol Misuse?* Yorkshire Addictions Research, Training and Information Consortium, York.

Mayo, M. (1994) *Communities and Caring*, Macmillan, Basingstoke.

Means, R. and Smith, R. (1994) *Community Care: Policy and Practice*, Macmillan, Basingstoke.

Mendes de Almeida, P.M. (1980) A review of focus group discussion methodology. *European Research*, **8**, 114–120.

Mermet, G. (1993) *Francospie: les Francais, qui sont-ils? Ou vont-ils?*, Larousse, Paris.

Middlemiss, C., Dawson, A.J., Gough, N. *et al.* (1989) A randomised study of a domiciliary antenatal care scheme: maternal psychological effects. *Midwifery*, **5**, 69–74.

MOH (1929) *Maternal Mortality in Childbirth Antenatal Clinics: Their Conduct and Scope*, HMSO, London.

MOH (1959) *Report of the Maternity Services Committee*, HMSO, London.

MOH (1970) *Domiciliary Midwifery and Maternity Bed Needs: The Report of the Standing Maternity and Midwifery Advisory Committee*, HMSO, London.

Morris, F., Head, S. and Volkar, V. (1989) The nurse practitioner: help in clarifying clinical and educational activities in accident and emergency departments. *Health Trends*, **21**, 124–126.

Mullen, P.M. (1991) Which market? The NHS white paper and internal markets, in *Markets, Hierarchies and Networks*, (eds G. Thompson, J. Frances, R. Levacic and J. Mitchell), Sage Publications/Open University, London.

Munro, S., Thomas K.L. and Abu Shaar, N. (1993) Molecular characterization of a peripheral receptor for canniboids. *Nature*, **365**, 61–65.

Murphy, D. and Rapley, C. (1986) Still living at home. *Community Care*, **622**, 25–27.

Murphy, E., Spiegal, N. and Kinmonth, A. (1992) 'Will you help me with my research?' Gaining access to primary care settings and subjects. *British Journal of General Practice*, **42**, 162–165.

Myerson, A. (1941) Review of *Mental Disorders in Urban Areas* by R.E.L. Faris and H.W. Dunham. *American Journal of Psychiatry*, **96**, 995–997.

National Audit Office (1992) *NHS Accident and Emergency Departments in England*, HMSO, London.

Nettleton, S. (1989) Power and pain: the location of pain and fear in dentistry and the creation of a dental subject. *Social Science and Medicine*, **29**, 1183–1190.

Nettleton, S. (1991) Wisdom, diligence and teeth: discursive practices and the creation of mothers. *Sociology of Health and Illness*, **13**, 98–111.

Nettleton, S. (1992) *Pain, Power and Dentistry*, Open University Press, Milton Keynes.

Nettleton, S. and Burrows, R. (1994) From bodies in hospital to people in the community: a theoretical analysis of the relocation of health care. *Care in Place*, **1**, 3–13.

Neundorfer, M. (1991) Coping and health outcomes in spouse caregivers of persons with dementia. *Nursing Research*, **40**, 260–265.

Nguyen-Van-Tam, J. and Baker, D. (1992) General practice and accident and emergency department care: does the patient know best? *British Medical Journal*, **305**, 157–158.

NHSME (1992) *Local Voices: The Views of Local People in Purchasing for Health*, NHSME, London.

NHSME (1993a) *The NHS Management Executive Business Plan 1993/4*, HMSO, London.

NHSME (1993b) *The Quality Journey: A Guide to Total Quality Management in the NHS*, NHSME, London.

Nieminen, H. (1986) Life circumstances and the use of mental health services: a five year follow up. *Social Psychiatry*, **21**, 123–128.

Nolan, M., Grant, G. and Ellis, N. (1990) Stress is in the eye of the beholder: reconceptualizing the measurement of carer burden. *Journal of Advanced Nursing*, **15**, 544–555.

NRHA (1992) *How Do We Create a Healthy North? Consultation on a Strategy to Improve Health and Health Care Across the Northern Region*, NRHA, Newcastle-upon-Tyne.

Oakley, A. (1981a) *From Here to Maternity: Becoming a Mother*, Penguin Books, Harmondsworth.

Oakley, A. (1981b) Interviewing women: a contradiction in terms, in *Doing Feminist Research*, (ed. H. Roberts), Routledge & Kegan Paul, London.

Oakley, A. (1982) The origins and development of antenatal care, in *Effectiveness and Satisfaction in Antenatal Care*, (eds M. Enkin and I. Chalmers), Heinemann, London.

Oakley, A. (1984) *The Captured Womb*, Blackwell, Oxford.

Oakley, A. (1985) Social support in pregnancy: the 'soft' way to increase birth weight? *Social Science and Medicine*, **21**, 1259–1268.

O'Brien, J. (1987) A guide to life style planning: using the Activities Catalogue to integrate services and natural support systems, in *The Activities Catalogue: An Alternative Curriculum for Youth and Adults With Severe Disabilities*, (ed. B.W. Willox and G.T. Bellamy), Brookes, Baltimore, MD.

O'Brien, J. (1992) Closing the asylums: where do all the former long stay patients go? *Health Trends*, **24**, 88–90.

O'Brien, M. and Smith, C. (1981) Women's views and experiences of ante-natal care. *Practitioner*, **225**, 123–125.

O'Flanagan, P. (1976) The work of an accident department. *Journal of the Royal College of General Practitioners*, **26**, 54–60.

Oliver, M. (1992) Changing the social relations of research production? *Disability, Handicap and Society*, **7**, 101–114.

Orr, J. (1980) *Health Visiting in Focus*, Royal College of Nursing, London.

Parker, G. (1990) *With Due Care and Attention*, Family Policy Studies Centre, London.

Paterson, B. and Bramadat, I.J. (1992) Use of the preinterview in oral history. *Qualitative Health Research*, **2**, 99–115.

Patrick, D.L, Scrivens, E. and Charlton, J.R.H. (1983) Disability and patient satisfaction with medical care. *Medical Care*, **79**, 1062–1075.

Patton, M.Q. (1990) *Qualitative Evaluation and Research Methods*, 2nd ed., Sage Publications, Newbury Park.

Pearson, P.H. (1988) Clients' perceptions of health visiting in the context of their identified health needs: an examination of process. University of Northumbria, PhD Thesis.

Pearson, P.H. (1991) Clients' perceptions: the use of case studies in developing theory. *Journal of Advanced Nursing*, **16**, 521–528.

Pease, R. (1973) A study of patients in a London accident and emergency department with special reference to General Practice. *Practitioner*, **211**, 634–638.

Peele, S. (1993) The conflict between public health goals and the temperance mentality. *American Journal of Public Health*, **83**, 805–810.

Pickin, C. and St Leger, S. (1993) *Assessing Health Need Using the Life Cycle Framework*, Open University Press, Buckingham.

Plamping, D. and Delamothe, T. (1991) The citizen's charter and the NHS. *British Medical Journal*, **27 July**, 203–204.

Platt Report (1962) *Accident and Emergency Services*, HMSO, London.

Plummer, K. (1976) *Documents of Life*, Allen & Unwin, London.

Pollock, L.C. (1986) An introduction to the use of repertory grid technique as a research method and clinical tool for psychiatric nurses. *Journal of Advanced Nursing*, **11**, 439–445.

Potter, J. (1988) Consumerism and the public sector: how well does the coat fit? *Journal of Public Administration*, **66**, 149–164.

Poulton, K. (1984) A measure of independence. *Nursing Times*, **22 August**, 32.

Prior, L. (1989) *The Social Organisation of Death: Medical Discourse and Social Practices in Glasgow*, Macmillan, London.

Prior, L. (1991a) Community versus hospital care: the crisis in psychiatric provision. *Social Science and Medicine*, **32**, 483–489.

Prior, L. (1991b) Mind, body and behaviour: theorisations of madness and the organisation of therapy. *Sociology*, **25**, 403–421.

Ranade, W. (1994) *A Future for the NHS? Health Care in the 1990s*, Longman, Harlow.

Rantakallio, P. (1979) Social background of mothers who smoke during pregnancy and influence of these factors on offspring. *Social Science and Medicine*, **14A**, 363–368.

Redding, D. (1991) Exploding the myth. *Community Care*, **893**, 18–20.

Reidy, M., Taggart, E. and Asselin, L. (1991) Psychosocial needs expressed by the natural caregivers of HIV infected children. *AIDS Care*, **3**, 331–343.

Richardson, A. and Ritchie, J. (1989) *Letting Go*, Open University, Milton Keynes.

Rittel, H.W.J. and Weber, M.M. (1974) *Dilemmas in a General Theory of Planning*, Petrocelli, New York.

Robinson, C.A. (1993) Managing life with a chronic condition: the story of normalisation. *Qualitative Health Research*, **3**, 6–28.

Robson, S. and Foster, A. (1989) *Qualitative Research in Action*, Edward Arnold, London.

Roche, S. and Stacey, M. (1986) *Overview of Research on the Provision and Utilization of the Child Health Services: Update One*, University of Warwick, Warwick.

Roderick, P., Victor, C. and Beardhow, R. (1990) Developing care in the community: GPs and the HIV epidemic. *AIDS Care*, **2**, 127–132.

Rodgers, E.M. and Shoemaker, F.F. (1971) *Communication of Innovation*, Free Press, New York.

Rogers, C.R. (1951) *Client-Centred Therapy: Its Current Practice, Implications and Theory*, Constable, London.

Rose, N. (1985) *The Psychological Complex: Psychology, Politics and Society in England 1869–1939*, Routledge & Kegan Paul, London.

Rose, N. (1986) Psychiatry: the discipline and mental health, in *The Power of Psychiatry*, (eds P. Miller and N. Rose), Polity Press, Cambridge.

Rosenhan, D. (1973) On being sane in insane places. *Science*, **179**, 1–9.

Roth, J. (1972) Some contingencies of the moral evaluation and control of clientele: the case of the hospital emergency service. *American Journal of Sociology*, **77**, 839–855.

Roy, A. (1987) Five risk factors for depression. *British Journal of Psychiatry*, **150**, 536–541.

Royal College of Nursing, Society of Primary Health Care Nursing (1983) *Thinking about Health Visiting*, RCN, London.

Sakala, C. (1989) Community based, community oriented maternity care. *American Journal of Public Health*, **79**, 897–898.

Salisbury, D. (1986) AIDS: psychosocial implications. *Journal of Psychosocial Nursing*, **24**, 13–16.

Saunders, P. and Harris, C. (1990) Privatization and the consumer. *Sociology*, **24**, 57–75.

Sbaih, L. (1993) Accident and emergency work: a review of some of the literature. *Journal of Advanced Nursing*, **18**, 957–962.

Scheff, T. (1966) *Being Mentally Ill: A Sociological Theory*, Aldine Press, Chicago, IL.

Scull, A.T. (1984) *Decarceration, Community Treatment and the Deviant: A Radical View*, Polity Press, Cambridge.

Sedgwick, P. (1982) *Psycho-Politics*, Pluto Press, London.

Shepherd, G. (1990) Case management. *Health Trends*, **22**, 59–61.

Sigelman, C. Budd, E. Spanhel, C. and Schoenrock, C. (1981) When in doubt say yes: acquiescence in interviews with mentally retarded persons. *Mental Retardation*, **19**, 53–58.

Silverman, D. (1985) *Qualitative Sociology: Describing the Social World*, Gower, Aldershot.

Simpson, M., Buckman, R., Stewart, M. *et al.* (1991) Doctor patient communication: the Toronto consensus statement. *British Medical Journal*, **303**, 1385–1387.

Skinner, B.F. (1972) *Beyond Freedom and Dignity*, Cape, London.

Small, R. Lumley, J. and Brown, S. (1992) To stay or not to stay: are fears about shorter postnatal hospital stays justified? *Midwifery*, **8**, 170–177.

Snaith, R.P., Ahmed, S.N. and Metha, S. (1971) Assessment of the severity of primary depressive illness. *Psychological Medicine*, **1**, 143–149

Social Services Committee (1982) *White Paper: Public Expenditure on the Social Services, Second Report from the Social Services Committee, Session 1981–2*, HMSO, London.

Soddy, K. (1962) *Cross Cultural Studies in Mental Health: Identity, Mental Health and Value Systems*, Quadrangle, Chicago, IL.

Spielberger, C.D., Gorusch, R.L. and Lushene, R.E. (1970) *Manual for the State-Trait Anxiety Inventory*, Consulting Psychologists Press, Palo Alto, CA.

Stacey, M. (1976) The health service consumer: a sociological misconception, in *The Sociology of the National Health Service*, (ed. M. Stacey), Sociological Review Monographs 22, University of Keele, Keele.

Stafford, J. (1993) Listen to local voices. *Maternity Action*, **59**, 9–10.

Straus, R. (1974) *Escape from Custody: A Study of Alcoholism and Institutional Dependency as Reflected in the Life Record of a Homeless Man*, Harper & Row, New York.

Strauss, A. (1987) *Qualitative Analysis for Social Scientists*, Cambridge University Press, Cambridge.

Strauss, A. and Corbin, J.M. (1988) *Shaping a Health Care System*, Jossey Bass, San Francisco, CA.

Strauss, A. and Corbin, J. (1990) *Basics of Qualitative Research*, Sage Publications, Newbury Park.

Strauss, A.L., Corbin, J., Fagerhaugh, S. *et al.* (1984) *Chronic Illness and the Quality of Life*, 2nd ed., CV Mosby, St Louis, MO.

Swain, J. (1993) Taught helplessness? Or a say for disabled students in school, in *Disabling Barriers: Enabling Environments*, (eds J. Swain, V. Finkelstein, S. French and M. Oliver), Sage Publications/Open University, London.

Symonds, A. (1993) Health visiting and the new public health. *Health Visitor*, **66**, 204–206.

Szasz, T.S. (1970) *Ideology and Insanity: Essays on the Psychiatric Dehumanization of Man*, Calder & Boyars, London.

Tajfel, H. (1982) *Social Identity and Intergroup Relations*, Cambridge University Press, Cambridge.

Tameside & Glossop Community Health Council (1987) *Primary Health Care Services*, Tameside and Glossop Community Health Council.

Taylor, S.J. and Bogdan, R. (1984) *Introduction to Qualitative Research Methods: The Search for Meanings*, John Wiley, New York.

Tew, M. (1990) *Safer Childbirth? A Critical History of Maternity Care*, Chapman & Hall, London.

Thomas, C. (1993) De-constructing concepts of care, *Sociology*, **27**, 649–669.

Thompson, C. (1989) London Lighthouse: a centre for people facing the challenge of AIDS, in *AIDS: Models of Care*, (eds M. Bould and G. Peacock), King's Fund/London Boroughs Training Committee, London.

Timms, N. and Mayer, J.E (1970) *The Client Speaks*, Routledge & Kegan Paul, London.

Tinker, A. (1984) Health and housing. *Nursing Times*, **80**, 18.

Tomlinson, B. (1992) *Report of the Enquiry into London's Health Service, Medical Education and Research*, HMSO, London.

Tones, K. Tilford, S. and Robinson, Y. (1990) *Health Education, Effectiveness and Efficiency*, Chapman & Hall, London.

Toohey, S. (1984) Parent–nurse interaction in the emergency department: an exploratory study. University of Alberta, Edmonton, PhD Thesis.

Toseland, R.W., Rossiter, C.M., Peak, T. and Smith, G.C. (1990) Comparative effectiveness of individual and group interventions to support family caregivers. *Social Work*, **35**, 209–217.

Townsend, J., Dyer, S., Cooper, J. *et al.* (1992) Emergency hospital admissions and readmissions of patients aged over 75 years and the effects of a community-based discharge scheme. *Health Trends*, **24**, 136–139.

Townsend, P. and Davidson, N. (1982) *Inequalities in Health: The Black Report*, Pelican, Harmondworth.

Townsend, P., Phillimore, P, and Beattie, A. (1988) *Inequalities in Health in the Northern Region: An Interim Report*, University of Bristol, Bristol and Northern Regional Health Authority, Newcastle upon Tyne.

Traynor, M. (1993) Some current issues for health visiting. *Health Visitor*, **66**, 216–218.

Treacher, A. and Baruch, G. (1981) Towards a critical history of the psychiatric profession, in *Critical Psychiatry*, (ed. D. Ingleby), Penguin, Harmondsworth.

Trostle, J.A. (1988) Medical compliance as ideology. *Social Science and Medicine*, **12**, 1299–1308.

Tudor Hart, J. (1971) The inverse care law. *Lancet*, **1**, 405–412.

Turner, B.S. (1993) Contemporary problems in the theory of citizenship, in *Citizenship and Social Theory*, (ed. B.S. Turner), Sage Publications, London.

Twigg, J. (1989) Not taking the strain. *Community Care*, **773**, 16–19.

Twinn, S. and Cowley, S. (1992) *The Principles of Health Visiting: A Re-examination*, Health Visitors' Association and United Kingdom Standing Conference on Health Visitor Education, London.

Tynan, A.C. and Drayton, J.L. (1988) Conducting focus groups: a guide for first-time users. *Marketing Intelligence and Planning*, **6**, 5–9.

Tyne, A. (1987) Shaping community services: the impact of an idea, in *Reassessing Community Health Care*, (ed. N. Malin), Croom Helm, Beckenham.

Tyrer, P. (1988) Dependence as a limiting factor in the clinical use of minor tranquillizers. *Pharmalogical Therapy*, **36**, 173–188.

Ungerson, C. (ed.) (1990) *Gender and Caring: Work and Welfare in Britain and Scandinavia*, Harvester Wheatsheaf, London.

Unschuld, P.U. (1986) The conceptual determination of individual and collective experiences of illness, in *Concepts of Health, Illness and Disease*, (eds C. Currer and M. Stacey), Berg, Oxford.

Van Teijlingen, E. and McCaffery, P. (1987) The profession of midwife in the Netherlands. *Midwifery*, **3**, 178–186.

Walker, R. (1982) An introduction to applied qualitative research, in *Applied Qualitative Research*, (ed. R. Walker), Gower, Aldershot.

Walmsley, J. (1993) It's not what you do but who you are: caring roles and caring relationships, in *Health and Welfare Practice*, (eds J. Walmsley, J. Reynolds, P. Shakespeare and R. Woolfe), Sage Publications/Open University, London.

Walsh, M. (1990) Geographical factors and A&E attendance. *Nursing Standard*, **5**, 28–31.

Warren, R. (1989) The other 99 per cent. *Health Service Journal*, **99**, 232–233.

Webb, C. (1984) Feminist methodology in nursing research. *Journal of Advanced Nursing*, **9**, 249–256.

West Birmingham Community Health Council (1990) *After an Accident: The Discharge of Elderly People from the Accident and Emergency Department of Dudley Road Hospital*, West Birmingham Community Health Council, Birmingham.

Westcott, G. (1987) The effects of unemployment on health in Scunthorpe and related health risks. *Public Health*, **101**, 399–416.

West Cumbria Community Health Council (1990) *A Survey of General Practice Patients' Views*, West Cumbria Community Health Council.

Which? Way to Health (1989) Your baby, your choice. *Which?*, **October**, 13–19.

Whitehead, M. (1987) *The Health Divide: Inequalities in the 1980s*, Health Education Council, London.

Whitehead, S. (1992) The social origins of normalisation, in *Normalisation: A Reader for the Nineties*, (eds H. Brown and H. Smith), Routledge, London.

WHO (1958) *The First Ten Years of the World Health Organization*, WHO, Geneva.

WHO (1980) *International Classification of Impairments, Disabilities and Handicaps: A Manual of Classification Relating to the Consequences of Disease*, WHO, Geneva.

WHO (1986) A discussion document on the concept and principles of health promotion. *Health Promotion*, **1**, 73–76.

Wiffin, A. (1993) Discharge procedures: are they effective in ensuring continuing care? Institute of Health Sciences, University of Northumbria, Postgraduate Diploma Thesis.

Williams, E.G. and Fitton, F. (1991) Survey of carers of elderly patients discharged from hospital. *British Journal of General Practice*, **41**, 105–108.

Williams, F. (1989) *Social Policy: A Critical Introduction*, Polity, Cambridge.

Williams, S., Dickson, D., Forbes, J. *et al.* (1989) An evaluation of community antenatal care. *Midwifery*, **5**, 63–68.

Williamson, V. (1988) *GP Services: Mothers' Views*, Brighton Community Health Council, Brighton.

Wilson, H.S. (1989) Family caregiving for a relative with Alzheimer's dementia: coping with negative choices. *Nursing Research*, **38**, 94–98.

Wistow, G. (1994) Community care futures: inter-agency relationships – stability or continuing change? in *Caring for People in the Community: The New Welfare* (ed. M. Titterton), Jessica Kingsley, London.

Wood, K.M. (1979) Nurse–patient communication in an accident department. University of Manchester, MSc Thesis.

Woolich, C. (1992) A wider frame of reference. *Nursing Times*, **88**, 34–36.

Yarde, M. and Forrest, A. (1989) *The Patients' Views of Services Provided by the Family Doctor*, Sheffield Community Health Council, Sheffield.

Zarb, G. (1992) On the road to Damascus: first steps towards changing the relations of disability research production. *Disability, Handicap and Society*, **7**, 125–138.

Index

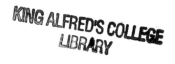